How to Help Your Child with ADHD

Practical ways to make family life run more smoothly

Beverly Davies

white
LADDER

Important note

The information in this book is not intended as a substitute for medical advice. Neither the author nor White Ladder can accept any responsibility for any injuries, damages or losses suffered as a result of the information herein. Anyone seeking advice on health should see their GP or appropriate health professional in the first instance.

How to help your child with ADHD: Practical ways to make family life run more smoothly

This first edition published in 2011 by Crimson Publishing Ltd., Westminster House, Kew Road, Richmond, Surrey TW9 2ND

British Library Cataloguing in Publication Data
A catalogue record for this book is available from the British Library

ISBN 978 1 90541 098 9

Typeset by IDSUK (DataConnection) Ltd
Printed and bound in the UK by Ashford Colour Press, Gosport, Hants

Thanks to everyone who helped with this book by telling me their story, and especially to Hugh

Contents

Introduction

ADHD stands for attention-deficit hyperactivity disorder. If you are the parent of a child with ADHD, this book is designed to help you help your child – from dealing with your initial worries and getting a diagnosis to smoothing a path through the ups and downs of family life. Above all, this book aims to make your child's life, and your own, easier and more fulfilling.

You might be very familiar with ADHD, and how it affects your child, or this subject might be totally new to you. Perhaps you've just discovered your child has ADHD, or strongly suspect he does.

The aim of the book is to inform you and, perhaps more importantly, to help you understand and communicate with your child better, so you can make a real difference to his life, and your family's. We take you through exactly what you need to know and include the stories of parents and children who have shared your experience. They tell you what they've found out the hard way – what works and what doesn't. We've also called upon various experts throughout the book to give their opinion and advice.

The need for information and understanding is paramount. A report from the World Federation for Mental Health (published in the National Institute for Health and Clinical Excellence (NICE) guideline, see p151 found that:

- 91% of parents questioned were often stressed or worried about their child's life
- 68% stated that their child with ADHD had been excluded from social activities because of their symptoms
- 61% said that family activities were disrupted
- 63% said their primary care doctor (general practitioner or GP) did not know much about ADHD
- 51% said the diagnosis took too long.

Children with ADHD find it very hard to concentrate, control their behaviour or focus their attention. They are likely to be restless, suffer from mood swings, general hyperactivity and poor co-ordination, say things on impulse and find a lot of social situations difficult. On the up side, they can have masses of energy and enthusiasm, which are great qualities when channelled in the right direction.

> 66 *He was always very chatty and very interested in everything and very interesting in what he had to say, but also kind of exhausting. He has always been good fun, and now that he is happier things are great. I think it is important to stress that there are positive aspects to ADHD, but sometimes you do have to seek them out.* 99
> *Hugh's mum*

ADHD first appears in early childhood, often becoming noticeable from about the age of two or three years, when it can be hard to decide if these characteristics are just annoying variations on normal childhood behaviour or a more serious problem. As a parent, you are the best judge, and if you have a feeling that it might be the latter it is in your child's best interests – and your own – to try to get a diagnosis, making your GP your first port of call. The condition can lead to problems at home and school, and affect your child's ability to learn and to get on with others. So the sooner you get some help with dealing with it the better.

> 66 *I love working with kids and I love being with kids and I thought that all the extra stuff I was having to do with Ben was just an extension of managing children. I put so much into it, and Ben did manage quite well when he was small, before we found out what was the matter, but the energy it required of me was massive. He has never been a nasty boy, or deliberately bad, but he can be completely exhausting, and for such a long time I felt I was dealing with everything on my own.* 99
> *Ben's mum*

It can be very painful to live with worries and uncertainty about your child. Not knowing whether his behaviour is normal or not, but feeling deep down that it probably *isn't* can make you feel very isolated. Getting a diagnosis should open the door to the help and support which will help him fulfil his potential, and will mean that the people he meets, including teachers, will understand the reasons why he behaves the way he does and, with any luck, will be more tolerant.

ADHD is one of those conditions that many people aren't very aware of – they have probably heard the term, but are unsure what it means or assume it is just a politically correct way of saying 'badly behaved'. Given that, it's hardly surprising that if your child has this problem, diagnosis can be elusive, especially as ADHD often occurs along with other problems. 'Naughty', 'lazy', 'disruptive' are labels that litter the educational path of many undiagnosed children with ADHD. Some parents are reluctant to access a diagnosis, and consequent treatment, because of the perceived stigma of a label, although for others being able to give a name to the problem turns out to be a positive thing.

> 66 For me it really helped a lot when I could put a label on it – knowing what it was gave me some hints of how to deal with it. Knowing was what I needed, but I can understand that some parents absolutely don't want that label. 99
> **Ben's mum**

Some parents have such a struggle to get to the bottom of what is wrong with their child that the diagnosis comes as a relief, though it is not often a surprise.

> 66 Whenever I talked to our GP, he used to put up his fingers in inverted commas when he used the word hyperactivity. It was such a put down. I felt that the subtext was that professionals thought it was just poor parenting, but he would do his best to help me. So

before I went back to the GP again I collected up loads of information and got together a file of things that matched Sally's behaviour. I saw a new GP who had just joined the practice and said we had had all these problems and it might be ADHD and she said she would investigate. It was such a comfort to feel that someone finally believed that our problems were real. 99
Sally's mum

People also argue over whether ADHD even exists, and the issue of ADHD medication is highly topical and controversial. Both sides of the argument can be equally persuasive – that ADHD responds to medication or it doesn't; that it is cruel to drug children or that it is cruel *not* to give them a chance of making the best of their schooldays by offering them treatment. When you have all the information, you have to decide where you stand. But it is likely that if your child shows signs of the condition you will be keen to do whatever you can to help him.

Critics of the use of medication are often ADHD-deniers, who would say 'For goodness sake, they are just naughty, what is wrong with that?' Arguably, these people will not have first-hand experience of a young child climbing up the panes of an upstairs sash window to get out through the little gap at the top, or the relentlessness of a child who simply doesn't get tired, or one who really, really cannot concentrate in school, even when he is trying his utmost. For parents whose children show behaviours like these, the naysayers certainly don't make things any easier.

Throughout the debate over medication, it's important to remember that it is not the only treatment, and it is recommended that other routes should be tried first. The focus of your decisions should always be what's best for your child. From the children interviewed for this book it is certainly possible to see that medication, carefully prescribed and used, can transform their lives. Hugh is about to go off to university, after having been all set to give up on school altogether, while Charlie, at primary school, has been able to get his thoughts down on paper in some sort of order for the first time, to his immense satisfaction. Hugh found sessions with a counsellor were very helpful; for Sally, excelling at sport helped her to get over some of her problems. We'll look at some of the alternative treatments in this book, as well as looking at how medication can help your child.

So, how do you chart your path through the minefield of ADHD? What do you need to know when you start? How much harder is it for your child to get to any given point on the educational map with ADHD? And will it affect his life forever?

Early intervention can make a crucial difference to the outcome for your child, and to how much he can enjoy and benefit from his schooldays. It's important to use all the channels available to you as a parent to get a diagnosis and some appropriate help, whether therapy, classes for you and your child or medication. Ask the professionals, starting with the school or nursery or your GP, and have a list of all your worries about your child and his behaviour with you to make things clearer. No one knows your child better than you.

> 66 At primary school Ben did very well because he is highly intelligent and he could do well without having to listen or concentrate and he was manageable behaviour-wise. I kept trying to say that despite this there was an issue, and I feel that if they had given me more credence and helped we wouldn't have had the issues we have got now he is a teenager. At primary school his work never seemed to trouble him because he would just get it over and done with very quickly so teachers would say they didn't think that was the problem. 99
> **Ben's mum**

ADHD can manifest itself from a very young age when a child cannot tell you how he feels. However, older children and teenagers can be very articulate about how it feels to have this condition – and even if they are not, their behaviour can spell out the way it makes them feel with sometimes hideous clarity. We'll give you some practical ways of handling your child's behaviour or frustrations throughout the book.

> ❝ Sally went into a more devious stage from about age four or five and I didn't feel she was always very honest with us. The stories were always totally implausible and always driven by this jealousy and frustration. Despite always wanting to be accepted and wanting to be liked she used to antagonise doctors because if they did try to help her she would behave so badly. ❞
> *Sally's mum*

> ❝ I think almost the worst part of it for Hugh before he got treatment was the frustration of knowing that he was at least as bright as his friends, if not rather more so, but was achieving much less than them and much less than his capability, which made him very frustrated and angry and had a very bad effect on his behaviour. Finding out that there was a reason for it and sorting that out has been the key to a much happier boy. Where he was getting very angry and threatening to leave school at 17 he is now about to go off to university with a clutch of good A levels. ❞
> *Hugh's mum*

ADHD can appear in different ways and become a problem at different stages of your child's life. But whether you are the parent of a girl, troubled from babyhood, or of a teenage boy who kept what he felt was a terrible secret for most of his schooldays, or of a bright boy who has thrown most of his chances away, the problems will be very real, and will almost certainly have impacted on the rest of your family. Throughout the book we aim to bring you support and advice that will make a real difference to your family and may just help you to change the course of the story.

Author's note

ADHD as used throughout the book also covers ADD (attention deficit disorder) and hyperkinetic disorder.

For consistency and ease of reading I have generally referred to all children as boys.

The information in this book has been approved by Holly Evans, ADHD Advisory Teacher at ADDISS.

Hugh's story

Hugh is a bright, charming, high-achieving 18-year-old boy from a high-achieving family, yet ADHD plagued him through most of his schooldays, to the point where he nearly walked away from his education altogether:

It is difficult to know when it really started. My earliest memory of things being a problem is of homework being really difficult to get on with. All little kids want to play and mess around, do anything but homework – that's normal – but when I knew I really had to get down to something in the quiet time in my room on my own, I just couldn't concentrate.

I remember cheating in my three times table test because I just couldn't get down to learning it, even though there were no distractions in my room then. I just sat there not doing it.

At school I was always a bit chatty and cheeky – and lots of lessons would start with everyone being like that and all very jolly and suddenly there would be the dreaded phrase 'Time to fill out the worksheet' and then everyone else would settle down abruptly to start work and I was still just looking around. I just couldn't concentrate and I would end up filling in silly answers and daydreaming. We would be going through practice exam papers and someone would say 'You have 10 minutes left' and I wouldn't even have started. That was a horrible feeling. Teachers thinking you are lazy when you can't understand why you can't get on with things. At that stage, if I tried to talk about it people thought I was just being silly and said I should just make myself do it. Everyone else flips a switch and is in work mode, and it is not so much that I can't flip the switch as that I don't really have a switch.

Slowly in my head the idea – which I didn't say out loud for fear of teachers being angry with Mum, or not believing me, or whatever – the idea of the word 'can't' was taking hold. My big sister said that no one likes doing work, and so I was nothing unusual and I must just make myself sit down and make myself get started like everyone else. So I was thinking, 'Well I don't think I'm special, I know nobody likes work', but I was trying really, really hard to make myself get on with things, and I felt that everyone else could do something that I just couldn't. That was probably the beginning of me being moody and slightly petulant. Teachers thought that I was just being lazy, and it still makes my blood boil to think about that now.

I did perfectly OK at school when it came to exams and things, but there was a dark feeling underneath. The best bit of the week was drama club, where for the first 20 minutes we would put on music and just dance. I could release all this energy and it was all about expression and emotion as opposed to this feeling of having to concentrate on the page in front of you. So I didn't talk to anyone about how I was feeling – I buried it. It wasn't a conscious thing. I suppose I maybe thought that everyone else was the same and I just got on with it.

Common entrance revision at 13 was horrible beforehand – it was a whole Easter holiday of feeling 'I can't do this', and I suppose that was the first time Mum and I talked about the idea that I found it hard to concentrate.

The idea of my having ADHD was kind of a standing joke amongst my friends. I just mentioned it once in a throw-away way about a year into secondary school and people leapt at it when I explained the acronym and they said 'That is you in a nutshell'.

I remember a teacher saying something like 'Hugh why are you doing that with the worksheet?' And I said, 'Oh I can't make myself write it, I think I have ADHD', and she said 'Oh, actually, I think you might.'

continued

continued from previous page

In my head that was a real eureka moment. For the first time in my entire life since the three times tables in year 2 and the constant feeling of finding things so hard and frustrating, to have this whole validation from just one throw-away comment was amazing. It was a glimmer of hope. Here was something that might give me a possibility of sorting things out, or at least an explanation. From there on I was straight on to the internet to find out more about it, and I certainly seemed to have most of the symptoms.

I raised the idea with Mum but it was just 'don't be silly', so for me that was back to square one. Now Mum knows more about it because she has read stuff, but then she didn't so you couldn't expect her to have spotted it. That was when all sorts of things were going on and I couldn't work out whether I was unhappy because things at home were a bit shaky or because of school work. I had got to the point before I got diagnosed where I was on the verge of dropping out of school. Without the help I got I don't think I would have taken my A levels – let alone got to university.

I got to the point where school was making me so unhappy that I wanted to leave. Mum begged me not to do anything rash and to think about a compromise. Then, when I said I really wanted to do something about the ADHD thing; that was the point at which she started to take it seriously. So after that long struggle we finally got there, but three years later than we could have.

Then things happened. Mum called up school and said I wouldn't be in for a week. I was so exhausted from basically two years of being unhappy and arguing with everyone – teachers and family and the situation just breaking down. We went to the GP, who referred us to a psychologist the next week.

Once you have letters from a psychologist and/or a psychiatrist confirming the condition, things change. At school once there was a label; suddenly, instead of getting mad with me, all the teachers were saying 'Oh, he can't do this, that's OK, give him time', and being really nice. So on the one hand it's an impetus to try really hard, be the best you can and confound the stereotypes, on the other hand it can be an excuse to be lazy and use it as a justification. As soon as people stop challenging you, you lose some of your reasons for trying.

The counsellor said why didn't I try just throwing myself into the system for one week, so I did every single bit of work exactly on time and I was never late for school and in assembly I sang the hymns and I tried to make myself interested in every little thing and that was just when I started the medication and wanted to devour information, and it carried on from there. That's when I got really into theatre and got so involved in stuff at school that I asked if I could board for the last year as I was there for pretty much everything except sleeping. I kept my scepticism about the place but I got as involved as possible. I was Mr Extra-curricular and I started a recycling society and geography society.

When I started having medicine, the first two weeks were probably the best time I have had at school in my entire life. The psychiatrist said to have 18mg of methylphenidate [also known as Ritalin]. There is only one dose that is lower than that. He said I shouldn't expect it to let me concentrate straight away and warned me not to see it as a miracle wonder cure. I would still have to put in the hard work.

The psychiatrist said that depending on how my body reacted I might feel like I had taken a recreational drug – euphoric, buzzy, with a fluttering in my chest – and that it takes some time for the body to adjust so I should take it every day for two weeks and report back. If it had been horrible and made me demented we would change it and if it did nothing to me we would change it. But I felt superhuman in those first two weeks before my body got used to it. I haven't taken it for ages now but after the first

continued

continued from previous page

two weeks whenever I took the medicine I didn't feel different at all, I just felt like me. It is an enabler.

Suddenly I could read a 350-page book in one sitting and not get up once, which was incredible for me. It was the first time ever that I had been able to finish a long book. I was just devouring information. I am thinking about the possibility of going back on medication for university. Since I stopped taking it I have noticed it has got more and more difficult to read a book. I don't want to be lazy and take the easy option but I do think I would benefit from taking it at university, at least in term time. I don't want to be just coping without it I want to be doing the best that I can do – and that means at this stage having the help of the medication. I don't want to go to university and only do three-quarters as well as I could, but I don't want to take it for life. I want to learn to control the ADHD for myself.

At school I took it for four months with no break at all. The longer you take it non-stop the more it tails off. I was mostly stopping in the holidays except before important exams. I don't want to get to university and for it to be a huge struggle because taking the medication at school has shown me that it doesn't have to be.

I feel really positive about what has happened. All the thinking that it has involved has made me more mature and more self-aware. People consistently think I am three or four years older than I am, whereas they always thought I was younger than I am before all this happened. I think I have done more self-analysis and thinking about what makes me tick than most people of my age probably have. I feel like I understand myself better than a lot of people my age understand themselves. I want to try to go on seeing a counsellor at university. If I hadn't reached that crisis point, which was horrible, I might well not have got to this stage, so it has really been a positive thing for me. I am much more confident of myself and my opinions.

Hugh's mum's experience

We first became aware of a problem when Hugh was about 11 or 12. He was clearly bright and seemed to be getting on fine in class, but was struggling to organise himself and to get things written down. There was a real mismatch between his obvious intelligence and what he was achieving.

When we took him to an educational psychologist, she did lots of tests – his IQ score was phenomenally high – 139 (genius is 140), while in other things he scored very low. She ruled out dyslexia and dyspraxia, but couldn't work out just what was wrong. He was doing OK but as he got further up the academic tree it was clearer and clearer that something was wrong, but we couldn't work out what.

Things got more and more difficult at home at around this time – we were in the early stages of getting a divorce, and things were getting worse for Hugh. He then self-diagnosed. He looked it up on the internet, being that sort of child, and he came to me and said he thought he had ADHD and could we do something about it. He was getting more and more unhappy, and more and more difficult, and wanting to leave school – it was the beginning of A levels by this stage and he had done alright in his GCSEs.

The psychiatrist we went to said that Hugh did have ADHD and he had probably always been able to cope with it until the extra stress brought on by the situation at home. Family problems combined with problems at school had pushed him to a point where he couldn't cope with it, and the psychiatrist's strategy was to treat Hugh by giving him a version of Ritalin with the aim of getting him to a point where he could cope again rather than it necessarily being a long-term prescription.

continued

continued from previous page

He stipulated to Hugh that there should be no recreational drugs – which you do need to spell out to a teenager – as they would really mess things up. He put him on a low-dose slow-release version of Ritalin. He said that what it does for someone like Hugh is to cut out the static that is buzzing round in his head, and Hugh finds that taking it really helps him to concentrate. Ritalin for most people is a stimulant but for Hugh it has the opposite effect, which is weird.

My take on it is that you have to try to find the positive side of any condition if you can. While Hugh has never been at the severe end of the spectrum, so I can't say it would be true for everyone, and I know you can't be glib with these broad-spectrum things because some people have a horrendous time, we certainly think there are positives.

1

What is ADHD?

ADHD comprises a range of problem behaviours, including impulsiveness, inattentiveness, restlessness and hyperactivity. Children with ADHD often have additional problems such as learning difficulties or sleep disorders. It should be stressed that ADHD itself has no effect on intelligence. Children with the condition are often very intelligent, creative and enthusiastic, and when their energy is directed constructively they can become high achievers. However, the problems of ADHD are often found to prevent children from learning and socialising well, and can cause difficulties both at school and at home.

> 66 Everyone else at school seemed to be able to just flick a switch from being chatty and lively to putting their heads down and getting on with work — and I couldn't. I would still be looking around. 99
> *Hugh*

Concentration difficulties make it hard for these children to learn at school, whatever their level of intelligence. The struggles they have can easily make them feel stupid or a failure, and low self-esteem is a key factor in ADHD. If nothing is done to help them, their education is bound to suffer. Not only that, but because their behaviour can make them very irritating to other children they can find it hard to make friends, and may feel lonely, unloved or disliked. It is a vicious circle that can lead some children to become more aggressive.

> 66 *Sally always wanted a best friend and to fit in. By the stage where you are choosing your own friends other children didn't gravitate towards her very easily. She often alienated them with her behaviour.* 99
> **Sally's mum**

A child with ADHD will often have other problems as well, such as non-compliant behaviour, aggression, learning problems, mood swings, clumsiness, immature language or motor tics. Young people and adults may be beset with tendencies to self-harm, a predisposition to accidents, substance misuse, delinquency, anxiety states or academic underachievement.

Related problems

It is not always the case, but a child may often have ADHD-related problems together with other conditions such as dyspraxia or autistic spectrum disorders, and a variety of other learning and behavioural disorders, in which case diagnosis can be very difficult. Some children also have anxiety or depression, Tourette's syndrome or bipolar disorder – at times the symptoms for ADHD and bipolar disorders can seem very similar, meaning it can be hard to differentiate between them.

Parents often talk about how hard it has been to unpick the problems caused by different strands in order to find the best ways of treating them. With time, and care, you should be able to find the best solutions for your child, and the good news is that a lot of research is going on and understanding of ADHD and related conditions is increasing all the time.

The science behind it

Research shows that the way the brain works in those with ADHD is different from people who do not have it. It is thought that neurotransmitters (chemicals in the brain that carry messages) do not always work properly in people with ADHD, that there is less activity in the parts of their brains that control activity and attention and there may be imbalances in the levels of certain chemicals, such as noradrenaline and dopamine. This is part of a combination of factors that can lead to ADHD, partially explained by the concept of 'executive function'.

Scientific studies have shown that people with ADHD can have abnormalities in some parts of the brain, including the prefrontal cortex, the area of the brain that's believed to control executive functions. As Dr Dan Rutherford explains: 'these include specific mental activities that allow self control, such as managing frustration, restraining outbursts, problem solving, memory recall, sustaining effort and focusing.' These will all be familiar as things that someone with ADHD finds very hard. The core symptoms of ADHD – hyperactivity, impulsiveness and inattention – may all arise due to problems with executive functions.

'The different levels of neurotransmitters may also have an effect on glucose levels in the brain, which affects activity in that area. Put simply, the more glucose used, the more energy and activity there will be in the brain. A study looked at glucose levels in adults who had been hyperactive since childhood and continued to have symptoms. It found that in people with ADHD, the areas of the brain that control impulses and attention used less glucose, which suggests they were less active. It has been suggested that if someone has lower levels of noradrenaline and dopamine, their brain can't make use of the glucose, so less energy is available to some parts of the brain, causing the symptoms of ADHD.'[1]

A study by a team from Cardiff University has suggested that ADHD is a genetic condition. These researchers claim that this gives strong evidence that the brains of children with ADHD are different from those of other children.

---

1   *From material by Dr Dan Rutherford GP (04.2007) on netdoctor.co.uk. Reviewed by Dr David Coghill, senior lecturer in family psychiatry.*

❝ We hope that these findings will help overcome the stigma associated with ADHD. Too often, people dismiss ADHD as being down to bad parenting or poor diet. As a clinician, it was clear to me that this was unlikely to be the case. Now we can say with confidence that ADHD is a genetic disease and that the brains of children with this condition develop differently to those of other children. ❞
Professor Anita Thapar, leader of Cardiff University's study into ADHD

ADHD cannot be cured, but it can be successfully managed with the right diagnosis and treatment, and symptoms often abate with age. There are different levels of ADHD – some children might suffer from morning until night, while others show symptoms only at some times of day, such as when they are feeling tired or angry. The level of ADHD your child shows will have a bearing on treatment, which could include an overhaul of diet and exercise, behavioural and family therapy and/or medicine.

The medications used for ADHD are 'psychostimulants'. Taking them helps children to focus their thoughts and ignore distractions. They are approved in this country for children aged six years and over, are thought to be between 70% and 80% effective and are used to treat ADHD which is moderate or severe. There is a risk of side-effects which should be explained to you, and your child will be carefully and regularly monitored. We'll go into more detail about medication in Chapter 3, and discuss whether it's right for your child.

What are the symptoms?

The symptoms of ADHD in a child fit into two sets of behavioural problems:

1. symptoms of inattentiveness
2. symptoms of hyperactivity and impulsiveness.

Symptoms usually fit into one of the three subtypes of ADHD:

a. mainly inattentive
b. mainly hyperactive-impulsive
c. combined.

Children with the inattentive type of ADHD, which may be called ADD, can't seem to get focused or stay focused on a task or activity. They are likely to be dreamy, disorganised types, who have an inability to concentrate or get on with things they need to do. They are more often girls and, as the condition does not draw attention to itself, are quite often undiagnosed.

Hyperactivity and impulsivity tend to go together. These children are always on the go (though this often calms down a bit as they get older). They act without thinking – running across the road without looking, or climbing to the top of tall trees and then having no idea how to get down; they are often surprised to find themselves in a dangerous situation.

Children with the combined type of ADHD, which is the most common subtype, have problems with paying attention, with hyperactivity and with controlling their impulses. This may sound like a description of the way all young children behave from time to time, but for those with ADHD this behaviour is the rule not the exception. It causes the child to have problems at home, at school and with friendships.

> 66 There is a feeling with ADHD that is described as a motor whirring away inside you that you can't control. I never, ever have my body all still, so there is always something moving and the longer I try and sit still and work the more that feeling of needing to move builds up until I want to explode. So I would time my work to the second and even if I was in the middle of writing a word, when the 20 minutes I had set myself to work were up there was just an explosion of relief and I would push the chair back, thinking 'that was horrible'.

It's like when you hold your breath for as long as you can and for a while there is a comfortable period and then it gets worse and worse, and then you finally breathe and it is such a relief. 99
Hugh

Hyperkinetic disorder is the name traditionally used in this country for the most severe version of ADHD, in which all types of symptom are present. It involves children who are very hyperactive, and impairs across all areas of life, and it is more than likely that it would need treatment with medication. It seems that nowadays most experts use ADHD as the term for all areas of the condition.

66 *I was always telling the GP that I was sure Sally was not right. I asked for something to help her sleep because the nights were awful but none of them would really listen they just said toddlers can be awful, this is nothing unusual. But when I could compare her to her brother, I realised just how different Sally was, how intense and driven. She could not sit back and take in what was going on around her. She had to be at the centre of it.* 99
Sally's mum

Symptoms usually start to appear when the child is a toddler, and always before the age of seven. If you are anxious, or your child's nursery or primary teacher mentions that they have concerns, it is best to visit your GP to arrange for an assessment by a paediatrician or psychiatrist. They will look, over a period of time, and in more than one setting, for various well-defined symptoms.

66 *The checklist I found showed that if you had two or more of this list of incredibly generic symptoms then you might have ADHD and you should think about seeing a psychologist. I scored a good 14 out of 15 – which is probably the best I've ever done in a test.* 99
Hugh

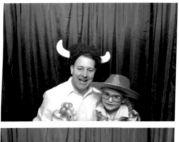

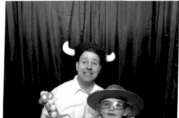

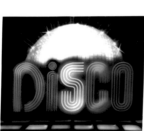

SPRING FLING 2014

Diagnosis of ADHD depends on strict criteria. Your child must have six or more symptoms of inattentiveness or six or more symptoms of hyperactivity and impulsiveness (see below). The type of ADHD a child is diagnosed with will depend on the number of symptoms he exhibits from each group. For instance, if he has, say, eight symptoms of hyperactivity and impulsiveness and three symptoms of inattentiveness, he will be diagnosed with ADHD mainly hyperactive-impulsive.

Your child must have been displaying symptoms continuously for at least six months, in at least two different settings – for instance at home and at school. This is to rule out the possibility that the behaviour is simply a reaction to particular teachers or to parental control. The child must have started to show symptoms before the age of seven, and the symptoms must make his life much more difficult on a social, academic or occupational level. The professional doing the assessment will want to make sure that the symptoms are not part of a developmental disorder or difficult phase, and cannot be better accounted for by another condition.

TIP In Chapter 2 we'll look at how you go about getting a diagnosis, and dealing with doctors and other health professionals.

Below is a list of symptoms of ADHD, relating to the different behavioural problems you might experience with your child.

Inattentiveness

Someone with inattentive symptoms of ADHD:

- has a very short attention span
- is very easily distracted
- seems forgetful and often loses things, and is disorganised about tasks and activities
- is unable to stick at tasks that are tedious or time-consuming
- is unable to listen to or carry out instructions

- is unable to concentrate
- fails to pay close attention to detail or makes careless errors during work or play
- fails to follow through instructions or to finish homework or chores
- avoids tasks that require sustained mental effort, such as homework.

Hyperactivity

Someone with hyperactive symptoms of ADHD:

- is unable to sit still, especially in calm or quiet surroundings
- is constantly fidgeting
- is unable to settle to tasks
- talks excessively.

Impulsivity

Someone with impulsive symptoms of ADHD:

- is unable to wait for his turn
- blurts out answers before the questions are finished
- acts without thinking
- interrupts conversations – butts into others' conversations and games
- breaks any set rules
- has little or no sense of danger.

> 66 *In the past he would do something silly and about half an hour later you would catch him crying and saying 'I don't know why I did that'. He just couldn't control himself.* 99
> **Charlie's mum**

> 66 *It wasn't just daydreaming it; wasn't just the normal thing where kids don't want to do homework. I would be all alone in the room with nothing else to do and a*

voice in my head asking 'Why aren't I just doing this?'
I just couldn't understand why I wasn't getting on
with it. 〟
Hugh

What does this behaviour actually look like?

Young children with ADHD sometimes seem like spinning tops of pointless and destructive activity. Parents describe them quite literally bouncing off the walls, being very aggressive and sometimes violent with siblings, hurling things off supermarket shelves. They just can't help it or do anything about it, but it can be upsetting for other people, and exhausting for the adults who have to try to calm them down – usually parents or teachers.

❝ *Charlie seemed to have a lot of temper tantrums around the age of three to four, he really started to seem different from the other kids. It was sometimes impossible to calm him down. He just couldn't ever sit still. Since he was little you have always had to keep him really occupied and grab his attention. When he started school he couldn't seem to understand about not wandering around the classroom or shouting out the answers to questions without putting his hand up and things like that.* 〟
Joan, Charlie's grandmother

FACT ADHD is a:

- developmental disorder
- found more in boys
- found in all social groups.

It may be:

- genetically linked – you may find other family members with the condition
- accompanied by other disorders
- associated with prematurity/smoking in pregnancy/being ambidextrous.

It is not:

- caused by bad parenting (though that can make it worse)
- caused by a poor diet, food additives or sugar (though they can make symptoms worse)
- caused by excessive television watching (though it is wise to limit this).

> 66 *I have never walked in a straight line with him, never in his life. Even now he is a teenager his friends say you can't go down a road with him without him stopping and starting and dodging about. The only time walking has ever been normal with him was when he was taking Ritalin and he would go in a straight line. It was completely different.* 99
> **Ben's mum**

The problems associated with ADHD can be seen in different ways at different ages, as the NICE guideline (p150) points out. A pre-school child who is hyperactive may be incessantly and demandingly active, at school age he may make excessive movements in situations where he might be expected to be calm rather than all the time, in adolescence this may become excessive fidgetiness rather than whole body movement, and as an adult it may translate into a sustained inner restlessness. Inattention may get less with age and attention span increase, but will still be less than the norm. It is, however, important to remember that many young people with ADHD will adjust well to adulthood and be free of mental health problems. This may be more likely when the main problem is inattention rather than hyperactivity-impulsivity, when antisocial conduct does not develop and when relationships with family members and other children remain warm.

66 *I have always been constantly on the move, but as I have got older I have realised that people get annoyed by my fidgeting around all the time. Try as I may it is impossible to keep still. One thing that has really helped is that I stopped trying to control my physical tics completely but by channelling all my constant activity into my toes I can conceal it a bit. Finding a physical tic that no one could see was quite important for me in terms of not feeling so noticeable. Accepting it and letting it happen actually calms it down. I used to feel very aware that my constant fidgety movement was unsettling for people, so this is much better.* 99
Hugh

ADHD and cultural norms

Personal cultural differences and expectations play a part in whether you think your child has ADHD, and they can vary a lot between individuals, let alone between nationalities.

66 *It is amazing how different people's views are of what is normal. A Japanese mother who came to my clinic thought her daughter had ADHD, and by the benchmarks of virtually any other culture she was one of the best behaved children I have ever seen, but by Japanese standards she wasn't able to sit in her Japanese lessons like the other Japanese children did. That is about cultural norms and expectations.* 99
Dr Dinah Jayson, Consultant Child and Adolescent Psychiatrist, specialising in neurodevelopmental disorders such as ADHD

This is why the diagnosis for ADHD is a complicated and time-consuming process (see Chapter 2). Health professionals must ascertain whether the behaviour could be dealt with by better parenting or needs further treatment, and is actually ADHD. This can be very frustrating if you feel that there are medical reasons for your child's behaviour.

Who gets ADHD?

Figures from the National Health Service (NHS) suggest that ADHD is the most common behavioural disorder in the UK. A recent estimate shows that up to 3 to 9% of school-aged children and young people are affected by the condition to some extent, with up to three times as many boys affected as girls. This may be because diagnosis tends to pinpoint the kind of loud, disruptive behaviour that is more noticeable in boys.

> **FACT** In a recent survey of 10,438 children age 5 to 15 ADHD was found in 3.62% of boys and 0.85% of girls.

Inheritance

The exact cause of ADHD is still unclear, but it is thought to be a mixture of genetic and environmental factors. It tends to run in families, and the condition is often thought to be inherited.

> **FACT** Research has shown that siblings and parents of a child with ADHD are four or five times more likely than normal to have the condition themselves.

Some recent genetic studies looking at inheritance patterns in families have shown that ADHD is one of the most heritable conditions. While genetic factors raise the risk of ADHD they don't dictate that the disorder will develop, and here environmental factors come into play.

> ❝ I am absolutely certain that I have ADHD too, which doesn't help, and makes being a mother quite difficult. There are a lot of hereditary factors. I never had any

diagnosis, it was just a feeling which came into focus when my daughter was diagnosed. 🙙
Daisy's mum

Pregnancy problems and prematurity

Children born prematurely are more likely than others to have developmental difficulties of various sorts, including ADHD, and there are potentially other factors relating to pregnancy and early environment that can have a bearing on the development of the condition.

🙙 *If the mother is very anxious during her pregnancy, high levels of stress hormones in the womb can increase the chances of ADHD if the child already has a genetic risk.* 🙙
Dr Dinah Jayson

Family circumstances and environmental factors

When a child's genes contain a risk of ADHD already, environmental factors can exacerbate and 'bring out' the condition.

🙙 *During childhood, some kind of disruption in the family home, or a lack of structured activities, support or supervision may contribute to problems in a child with a genetic tendency to ADHD. This is not about bad parenting, but sometimes the environment that provides the chance for ADHD to develop is due to circumstances such as where you live, a lack of support or an illness.* 🙙
Dr Dinah Jayson

Charlie's story

Charlie is seven years old and has recently started to take medication for ADHD, which has been a problem for him since he was two. He lives in Newcastle with his mum, Lisa, and two younger siblings. Granny Joan lives nearby. A busy single mum, juggling the needs of three children and a part-time job, Lisa is delighted that the changes brought about by the medication have made Charlie much happier:

There was always something about Charlie. Even during the terrible twos he had that extra bit of spark and personality about him, and he could be really impossible. I took him to the doctor a lot but they said that even if there was anything wrong they wouldn't do anything when he was that young. They finally diagnosed him a month ago, aged seven. From when he was about two I would sit down after he had gone to bed and just cry because I was so exhausted by trying to deal with him all day. I really struggled with him, and it affected my relationship with his little brother's father because I was so drained. It wasn't Charlie's fault but it was a major factor because we would argue because he was so wild.

His school recognised that he had problems, and finally it was the headmistress who did his referral and then we spent over a year going to CAMHS [Child and Adolescent Mental Health Services] before his actual diagnosis, so no one could accuse them of rushing. The health worker came to do his assessment at school. He has had the psychological tests and tests to rule out other conditions and has been observed in the school setting, and even though he was always so hyper and loud, everyone who has assessed him has remarked on what a lovely boy he is. When he had the observations in school, the woman who assessed him was amazed because he went to get his lunch box and started offering her biscuits and things, and at the end he hugged her and thanked her.

He is just different and he stands out from the other kids. He is soft and gentle a lot of the time, but he is like a puppy jumping around all the time. He is a boy who can be polite, caring and careful of others when he is not going mental.

He is on methylphenidate now, and it has made a major difference. The day after he first started taking it was his baby sister's first birthday party. Normally at something like that I am constantly having to tell him off because he is zooming around at 100 miles an hour, and in that sort of situation it has always been a nightmare. This was the first time that I didn't have to say anything to him at all. Everyone who knows him has noticed the difference.

Since he has had the medicine it has been different, but in the past if you took him out everyone would be staring and he was really wild. He is still fidgety, but nothing like as bad. With his school work he is a whizz at maths and creative work and he is advanced in those, but things like English, where you have to sit and learn things, or write them down, have been problematic. Normally if they were trying to write a story in English which needs a beginning, middle and end, he would just blurt out masses of ideas to the teacher in a random order, because he just couldn't get it organised in his mind and he would get so frustrated because he couldn't write it down. I had a meeting recently with the teacher and she brought a couple of bits of work that he had sat down and done on his own. For the first time ever he had really taken his time and concentrated, and the letters were all the same size, and there was even punctuation. That is a massive achievement for him and he is noticing that he is getting praise and noticing that it is better to behave.

The school was putting a bit of pressure on me to up his medication, but I am reluctant to do that at the moment . . . I think he is still getting used to it and he has had a lot of uncertainty to deal with about who was giving him his lunchtime

continued

continued from previous page

tablets, as it has been lots of different people so far. Routine is very important to him, and I think he will settle down much more once that is all sorted out. He really needs the stability of knowing when and where everything will happen in his day and he is settling down into it. If he doesn't know where something is or something changes in his routine it can send him right up the wall. I have noticed a massive change in him already at this level of medication and I want to give him a few more weeks of school to prove that he can settle down before we have to think about upping the dose.

In the past, unless we had a planned day out I would never take Charlie out with me. If I had to go into town or to the supermarket I would have to get someone to come in and watch him. I can't count how many times I have just had to walk out of the supermarket and leave my shopping in the aisle because Charlie was running around madly. We would go out and everybody would be staring and saying 'Can you not control your child?' and there he would be spinning round on the floor and throwing stuff.

It has affected my relationships in the past, it has affected friendships where people haven't wanted their kids anywhere near him because he was so wild sometimes, it has affected our whole lives. I was doing really well at work when he was small and of course he comes first so I had to cut down my hours because he needed me. Obviously I don't begrudge it at all, but it has had consequences.

To celebrate how well things are going with the medicine I gave him a surprise and we went out to the pictures and for dinner, just the two of us for a treat. So I picked him up from school and we went to the bus stop and I didn't think the driver would let us on the bus because he had chucked us off before when Charlie had behaved badly and I could see him thinking 'Oh here we go again'. Charlie just sat down and said, 'You sit next to me Mummy', and sat there good as gold all the way into town.

We went for some dinner and in the past it has been sauce everywhere and him running around and we usually ended up taking the food out with us – but this time he sat down and set the table and behaved nicely all through the meal, and then sat throughout the film and said 'Thank you' to the usherette at the end. After our outing, I sat down when Charlie had gone to bed and just cried because I couldn't believe how different he was. I've always known that he is a good boy, and people who really know him have always understood that he has a heart of gold – it is just people who don't know him have always looked at him differently as if he is a bit loopy. It is so refreshing to see him feeling so much better about himself and I feel really positive about it.

2

Getting a diagnosis

Dealing with doctors and experts

The time before diagnosis, when you are sure that something is wrong, but can't be sure what it is, can be wretched for parents. The condition can lead to problems at home and school and affect your child's ability to learn and to get on with others, so the sooner you get some help with dealing with it the better. But where should you start?

Where to start

As a parent, you are the best judge, and if you feel something's wrong, make your GP your first port of call. Your GP will give your child a medical examination, ask about his medical history, and check his vision and hearing to rule out other possible causes.

There is no simple test for ADHD and if your GP thinks that ADHD is possible, it is likely, and preferable, that he or she will arrange for your child to see a paediatrician, or child psychiatrist for assessment. This will involve observing your child over a period of time in at least two different situations – for instance, home and school, and the observations will be based on a variety of criteria and questions.

A child must display at least six of the symptoms listed on pXXX for at least six months before an official diagnosis of ADHD can be given, so the process will take *at least* six months, and probably longer. It needs to take this long as it would be impossible to say whether or not a child had the condition based on a single behavioural trait and a brief examination over a short period of time. However, many parents find this process worryingly long, especially if they have left it a while to seek medical help. It is six more months of not knowing for sure whether your instincts match up with the professionals.

TIP If you are just embarking on the road to diagnosis, keep a notebook handy and write down all the instances your child has displayed any of the symptoms on p21–22. This will come in very handy at your first appointment, as you may struggle to remember the best examples of your child's behaviour.

An alternative route towards diagnosis is through your child's school or nursery, as teachers are often the first to notice signs of ADHD. They can refer your child via CAMHS or suggest to you that you proceed yourself via your GP or one of these services. They will also have access to advice from an educational psychologist.

66 *His behaviour in the classroom was deteriorating, and he couldn't seem to stop wandering around the classroom or shouting out the answers to questions without putting his hand up. The headmistress had a word with his mum because his behaviour was having a knock on effect on the class, and the school referred*

*him on to the child mental health team. They came
and sat in on some of the lessons and did tests
with him.* **"**
Joan, Charlie's grandmother

The steps of assessment

The NICE guideline on the treatment of ADHD within the NHS
recommends that assessment includes the following.

1. A clinical interview: this is carried out by a paediatrician,
   psychiatrist, clinical psychologist or specialist nurse, and the
   aim is to detail the full range of the problems and their history,
   as well as family health, social and educational information.
   It should take two to three hours, often spread over two
   interviews, and involve the child and parents, separately and
   together, and maybe other involved parties such as teachers.
2. A medical examination: this is undertaken by a paediatrician or
   psychiatrist with the aim of ruling out undiagnosed disorders
   such as hearing impairment, epilepsy and some genetic
   conditions, plus co-existing disorders such as dyspraxia or sleep
   disorders. If a diagnosis of ADHD is confirmed, and drug therapy
   considered, the examination will include baseline measurements
   of height, weight, blood pressure, pulse rate, as these can be
   affected and will be monitored throughout treatment.
3. Observation in educational and domestic settings and other
   assessments such as developmental and literacy skills.

All this needs to be carried out over a period of time to ensure an
accurate picture is obtained.

> TIP You may be surprised by the lack of awareness
> and recognition of ADHD symptoms both among
> healthcare professionals and in schools. Often, action has to
> be driven by parents who have researched the condition or
> realise that their child may have a problem.

How old must my child be to get a diagnosis?

While you may suspect ADHD from a very early age in your child, diagnosing a pre-school child can be very difficult. If a child is behaving badly there is pretty much always a reason, it's just that the reason can be any number of things, and ADHD is only one of them. There are many conditions with similar symptoms, such as developmental disorders and some learning disorders, and a lot of children will have symptoms of ADHD simply by virtue of being young – such as running around manically or refusing to sit down for five minutes or blurting out things they didn't mean to say. But if you can't find a simple explanation at home, such as family problems or a lack of discipline, and a teacher can find no obvious explanation at school such as dyslexia or boredom-induced bad behaviour in a bright and under-stimulated child, then it is time to ask an expert, starting at the GP surgery with the aim of being referred onwards.

> 66 If diagnosis is left later, parents can be getting blamed for being bad parents and that is just destructive. Being attacked every day as a parent when what you have is a difficult kid is not going to help you. We want to try to manage things better so that we get informed referrals from as young an age as possible. 99
> **Dr Dinah Jayson**

The NICE guideline states that six years is the youngest age suitable for ADHD medication, but this does not mean diagnosis has to wait until then. The optimal age for diagnosis is simply *as early as possible*, so referral might realistically start to happen from three or four years of age. You may find that your child's ADHD has become much more noticeable as he starts nursery or school, and can less and less easily be put down to excitement or 'children being children'.

66 *He will just blurt out the most ridiculous things. He has always been like that. When he was little he was called a tell-tale at school a lot because he would always tell the teacher what the others were doing. He would see what someone was doing and go 'Oh look they are drawing on the table' with no thought about whether he should say it or not. It is really say what you see with him, and it turned out that that is just part of the whole ADHD thing.* **99**
Ben's mum

Perseverance is key

As a parent, it is important to make sure that your child is properly assessed. The length of time that it should take to get a diagnosis of ADHD shows that the condition is being taken seriously. No one wants to give medication unnecessarily, or if it is not the right medication, and it is important to establish exactly what is wrong. As this is a condition that involves behaviour, the behaviour has to be looked at by people who understand it in order for a judgement to be made. Therefore, try to bear with what can feel like an incredibly long process, full of hoops to jump through. Health professionals are trying to ensure they do what's best for your child, and giving a wrong diagnosis of ADHD, when it may be a myriad of other things (see p16), does not help anyone.

That said, perseverance when getting a diagnosis is essential. If you or your child's teachers have been sufficiently concerned to go to a GP as a start in the process of diagnosis, try to make sure things don't end there, with a quick check-up and a prescription. In this condition each diagnosis is very individual and there is benefit to be gained from non-medical treatments, which should be tried before you look at medical ones. It is only fair to your child to explore all possibilities, and proper assessment by trained professionals is the recommended route.

TIP Try to ensure you are referred onwards from your GP, to a paediatrician, psychologist or CAMHS. Where services are overstretched you may feel the waiting time for an appointment is very long. If so, it might be worth getting in touch with your local Patients Advisory Liaison Service (PALS).

Health professionals – who's who

- GP: Your first port of call, he or she will refer you on to specialists or CAMHS.
- Paediatrician: A doctor who is an expert in the health and development of children, and can assess whether problems are due to physical or emotional causes.
- Educational psychologist: A specialist who has studied how children learn and behave. Every school in the UK should have access to a free educational psychologist service, accessed through the local education authority.
- Child psychiatrist: A doctor trained to diagnose and treat a wide range of psychiatric disorders and illnesses in children and young people.
- CAMHS: In every area the health service has specialist child psychiatrists, psychologists, psychotherapists, social workers and mental health nurses, who work in multi-disciplinary teams to help children and their parents understand and deal with mental health problems and disorders.

Your first appointment with the doctor

Before your initial appointment, write down all the troubling symptoms your child is displaying or has displayed and which have caused you to seek medical help. Take these notes with you so that you can discuss them. Any information you can give them about everyday things such as sleeping and eating problems, behaviour at home, at nursery or school and when out and about, and any health concerns you have will help put the doctor in the picture.

The doctor will also ask you whether there are any circumstances at home that might be affecting your child, and also your family's medical history. Has anyone else had similar problems? It can all be relevant, and writing everything down beforehand will make sure that you don't forget something in the stress of the appointment. If you can, make a double-length appointment so that you do not have to feel rushed.

> **TIP** Tell your child why you are going to the doctor and see what he thinks about it. Does he understand why you are going to the doctor, and that they may ask him some questions?

During the appointment, it is a very good idea to make notes of everything that the doctor tells you, or take your partner or a friend with you to do so while you listen and answer his or her questions. If you get too much information all in one go, something important can easily slip your mind.

Don't feel it's your job to persuade the doctor your child needs to be assessed. Try to go in with a clear head, and your 'evidence' written down succinctly.

> 66 I used to find that I would take him to the doctor and the hospital and that was the only time he would sit quietly, which probably made them think I was making a fuss about nothing. 99
> **Charlie's mum**

Should I bring my child?

You may not have thought of this, but many parents find that attending the initial appointment without their child is a lot easier. You can explain your worries openly, without your child having to listen to conversations about his behaviour. He may not understand why he acts the way he does, so hearing adults discussing it could be even more upsetting. Once you've had a preliminary chat, you can then bring your child back for the doctor to meet him and ask him some simple questions.

Questions your doctor may ask you

- Do you have any family history of ADHD or other behavioural difficulties?
- What is your child's behaviour like on a daily basis?
- Are there any times when you notice his behaviour gets worse?
- Does he find it hard to concentrate or sit still for any length of time?
- How do you and your partner deal with bad behaviour?
- Is there anything going on at home that could be contributing to his behaviour?
- What is your child's diet like, and sleeping patterns?
- If he has started school, have any teachers commented to you on his behaviour?

Questions to ask your doctor

- How can you be sure it is ADHD and not something else?
- Does my child need to have medication, or are there alternative treatments?
- What are the risks associated with medication? How does it work?
- How long will my child have to take medication, and will long-term use hurt him?
- If I have other children, what is the likelihood that they will have ADHD too?
- Will my child grow out of ADHD or will he have it for life?
- What support will my child need – at school and at home?
- What support can you give me and where can I find out more?

Your initial meeting with your GP is likely to lead to your child bring referred to other health professionals for further assessment tests. If you are convinced that your child may have ADHD but your GP does not want to investigate it you can request to see another GP.

If you try this, and get the same response but strongly feel it may be ADHD, you could arrange to see an educational psychologist privately for an independent assessment (see p46). Armed with a report, you may find it easier to be referred into the appropriate channels.

> **TIP** A very good source of information at this stage is YoungMinds, the children's mental health charity (www.youngminds.org.uk) You can find out more about the help that is available and how to access it by contacting the YoungMinds parents helpline on 0808 802 5544.
>
> You can also get help and information from the Attention Deficit Disorder Information and Support Service (ADDISS; www.addiss.co.uk).

What happens after referral?

Referral should lead to a full specialist assessment where your child's needs will be clearly identified. The pathways vary around the UK, as does what will be offered to you, but the next step will generally be an appointment either with a specialist paediatrician or with a child psychiatrist, or you may be referred to CAMHS. Your child could also get referred to an ADHD assessment centre, which would include assessments by paediatricians, psychologists and school visits. The whole process of assessment will probably take at least six months, and it can take a while to get the referral appointment booked in too.

The specialists will need to know your child's medical, family and psychiatric history and your detailed account of his problems (so bring your notes again). Sometimes you will be sent a detailed questionnaire on development and behavioural matters before the appointment.

The specialist will do a physical examination to rule out an underlying medical cause for the problems and may then order further tests, and may use physical tests to assess motor skills, such as testing your child's ability to write, or catch a ball. Other tests may check his ability to understand what is said, and to express himself. Details on your child's educational history, illustrated by comments from the teacher or school, may be asked for, and depending on what these say, they could lead to a more formal assessment by an educational psychologist.

> **TIP** As the artificial environment of a clinic can make your child behave untypically (either better or worse) the specialist will sometimes arrange to see them in another setting such as home or school, before making a diagnosis.

If you are to be seen by CAMHS, the services offered vary around the UK, so you will not necessarily know what to expect or who you will see at your appointment. To set your mind at rest before you and your child go for your first appointment you can ask the CAMHS secretary to send you some information about how it all works at your local CAMHS, or to talk you through it on the phone. This will be reassuring for your child as well.

At the appointment you will benefit if you take a list of the problems your child has been having, when they started, if there is a pattern to the behaviour, any difficulties in school or with friendships, past and present health problems and any significant family events or traumas.

Make sure your child has a chance to speak up, and also, if there are things about your child that you are reluctant to discuss while he is there, try to have an additional discussion on your own.

Don't be afraid to ask as many questions as possible during your appointment, such as what the diagnosis will mean for your child, how severe the problem is, what treatments there are and whether lifestyle changes could reduce the need for other treatment or medication. Writing down questions before can make it easier to cover all the ground you want to in your allotted timeframe. See p40 for some suggestions.

Effective treatment will include advice and support for the parents. You should be able to expect the following:

- a full explanation of the condition to you and your child
- advice on how to manage difficult behaviour
- communication between the child's specialist and teachers
- advice on structured activities and reward systems for positive behaviour
- advice on special support and teaching if needed
- help for difficulties that have developed as a result of ADHD, such as low self-esteem and difficulty with friendships, temper tantrums and aggression.

If the specialist diagnoses your child as having ADHD, they will then suggest treatments. The most obvious of these is, of course, medication, but there are other treatments to consider, which may work well for your child. Make sure you're aware of the different treatment methods available, so that you can ask your specialist which ones they would suggest, besides going down the medication route. We'll look at treatments in detail in Chapter 3.

66 *It takes a minimum of six months to get the diagnosis. Then in general the result in my experience is that the only thing they offer is medication. In my work running the ADHD support group for some years now my son and most lads like him would run a mile rather than having anything like cognitive behavioural therapy [CBT] – but it would be nice to be offered. They tend to deal with everything with medication and/or lectures to the parents. Parenting courses are not routinely offered by any means but parents sometimes get referred to courses by Barnardo's. The problem can be that there are very basic things suggested – a lot of it is common sense. Sometimes, though, just being told that it is*

because of something in your child's brain, that he is not doing it on purpose and it is not really his fault, or your fault, can help you to get it into perspective. 🔊
Billy's mum, who runs an ADHD support group

TIP Treatment options for children and their families are inconsistent around the country, the treatments themselves vary in different areas, and are provided in different settings, including specialist CAMHS or paediatric clinics. Ask your GP and specialists exactly what will be available to you in your area, so you are clear about the options.

Why diagnosis is important

'There are some people out there – professionals included – who are very judgemental one way or the other – they just have a very black and white view of things that are not very black and white,' says Dr Jayson, whose years of experience with this condition have led her to appreciate the complexity of both the causes and the effects of ADHD within a family. 'In some situations there is a lot going on and for children who really have a significant problem in this area, and their families, if they don't get the support and recognition and treatment they have got an outcome that is really appalling. This is borne out by the criminal statistics, the drugs, alcohol, accident statistics; lots of really serious outcomes that are directly related to untreated ADHD, which is a treatable condition.'

🔊 *I am a GP and I have patients with this stuff and a lot of them haven't even managed to get on the bottom rung of the ladder. The kids are climbing round my surgery and I'm thinking they probably have ADHD but nobody has even mentioned it. They are just in*

*trouble at school. Some of these children don't get the
help they need at school; they fall by the wayside, and
then what happens to them? You only have to go round
looking at the young offenders' institutions and they
are full of them. I think we should be making an effort
at a much younger level than we are and thus averting
all kinds of problems later.* 🍂
Daisy's mum

Summary of what should be looked at in assessment

The assessment of ADHD is made by looking at key characteristics:

- inattention, hyperactivity and impulsivity
- the inappropriateness of these characteristics when compared with other children at a similar developmental level
- symptoms that have been present for some time
- difficulties seen in more than one setting, for instance both home and school
- an adverse impact on development and social adjustment.

Those making the assessment will bear in mind that:

- ADHD may co-exist with other learning disabilities and cognitive problems as well as other mental health problems
- assessment should consider whether ADHD is the sole cause of impairment or whether other mental and physical disorders or personal and social circumstances are contributory factors
- there is no single, definitive psychological or biological test for ADHD
- diagnosis will be the outcome of several strands of investigation and this will require co-operation between a number of professionals working in different areas.

66 *The psychiatrist was, I felt, the first legitimate professional I had encountered. He challenged me as to whether I was just moulding myself around the symptoms of ADHD I had read about online or whether I actually had them. He had all my school reports from the very beginning and said that, whatever the problem, I had clearly always coped with it and passed exams and so on, so what was the problem now? He thought that family stuff had pushed me over the coping level. The more I saw him the more I realised that his way of helping me was to challenge me. He would make me get angry and tell him what I felt in just a sentence. And that helped me to understand what I felt.* 99
Hugh

The role of the educational psychologist

A consultation with an educational psychologist is often suggested after referral from a GP or your child's school. So, what can you expect when you go for your first appointment?

66 *Before the educational psychologist sees a client there has often been a conversation between the parent and the school, and the school may well initiate the interview. They may feel that they have done everything they can and they need someone else to join in with the problem solving. A psychologist's role is to help people solve problems, to act as a bridge between the parents and the school, so what we do is use our psychology to get parents and schools talking together and looking at the child in the class, in the playground and at home and putting all the pieces of the puzzle together to work out what is going on with the child, and what is contributing to the behaviour*

that is seen as a problem by parents and teachers. It is very much a collaborative problem-solving exercise between the parent, the school and the external specialist, also sometimes a paediatrician.

If I have been contacted by a school I would then have an initial meeting with the parent and the school together. If I am having a consultation with the parent, they will come in with the child, and I will see them both separately. First a 30–40 minute interview with the parent. If the child is deemed a young adult, which can be as young as 12 depending on their ability and the issues involved, they may well be included in that meeting, otherwise the child will be in the waiting room and then I will see them for one to one and half hours with short breaks. While I am working with the child, I would get the parents to fill in some questionnaires and developmental checklists. That provides a snapshot of behaviour over the last month and then will be considered along with other observations, because the clinical criteria are that the child's problem behaviours have been long-standing, so of more than six months' duration.

At the end of the consultation I debrief with the parent so that they can ask any questions and we can have a little chat about the way forward. In total it is about a three to a three and a half hour session. Sometimes that is done at the school, and that can be advantageous because you then have the school view right from the initial interview. I always give people the option of having a separate, one-to-one [interview]. Sometimes there will be things that the school wants to discuss privately as well.

I put all the information together in a written document and try to answer the questions: What is stopping this child from doing XYZ? How severe are those road blocks? What are some practical ideas for school and home to think about?

Being cautious most psychologists start off with a family and school behaviour management programme. With ADHD that is about having clear rules, a clear line of command, so he knows who is in charge, clear boundaries and structures and consistent consequences for actions. Classroom things like work stations, removing distractions, breaking things into short chunks, using egg timers.

I work closely with paediatricians and when the problems merit it – if a child has major difficulties with attention control or impulse control – I would then refer to a paediatrician for a full paediatric assessment.

When it is in the context of a local authority recommendation, . . . [educational psychologists] see children and parents much more regularly and often we will see a child for five years or so, therefore the reports are shorter. In the private sector, we will usually only see the child once or twice so the reports are much more comprehensive because they need to provide all the information for long-term reference. I will occasionally be involved in a further planning meeting after that and set up a programme which I monitor with the school. Normally I would make the recommendations and the school and family would implement them. **"**
Jeremy Monsen, Educational Psychologist

If you were not referred by your GP, you may want to book in another appointment to show them the educational psychologist's assessment. This may be enough to persuade them to refer you to other specialists.

3

Treatment methods and medication

While popular opinion in much of the media suggests that GPs are dishing out Ritalin like Smarties, most children with ADHD are treated with behavioural strategies as a first line, and in many areas parents are likely to be offered parenting courses to ensure that they have the right techniques to cope with the challenging scenarios involved in caring for a child with ADHD before medication is even considered.

Medication usually only comes in when the child is so affected by the condition that it is impairing his ability to learn, and NICE guidelines suggest that it is never prescribed before the age of six, and is only prescribed after extensive assessment. So, even if you think that medication is the way forward it will probably be at least six months before you have a prescription, and then only if your child meets the age criterion.

66 *Sally was six and I was concerned about any sort of mind-altering drugs, but we were pretty much at our*

wits' end. The doctor gave us confidence that she knew what was wrong and she could help as opposed to 'Just try this and see what happens'. Also, the research I had done confirmed that Ritalin was the answer and I suppose in my mind I had wanted that diagnosis. 🙶
Sally's mum

Chapters 4–6 contain specific advice on what you as parents can do to help your child – be that through parenting strategies or through dieting and exercise. First we'll consider some of the therapies that we know other parents have found helpful. Have a look through these, and discuss any with your GP that you feel may suit your child.

Therapies

Counselling

Counselling is provided by people who are trained to listen carefully to children's problems without criticising them, so they can talk about their worries and feelings and learn how to manage them. Counsellors don't give advice, but help children to decide things for themselves. You may wonder what your child will say, but, for it to work, you need to let your child know that he has your approval for talking to the counsellor, and you will know that the strict code of professional ethics includes confidentiality.

If your child consents, the counsellor may meet you periodically to discuss progress, but some children, and more especially teenagers, may want to keep things private. Many counsellors work for fixed periods of appointments such as six to 12 weeks.

The school or your GP should have details of local counselling services for children, and such services are sometimes available in schools, youth clubs or advice centres and sometimes, but not always, at your local CAMHS. Check that your child's counsellor has accreditation from the British Association for Counselling and Psychotherapy (BACP; www.bacp.co.uk).

Psychotherapy

Psychotherapy is in many ways similar to counselling, and similar skills are used. The process of psychotherapy may take longer and involve greater exploration of past experiences. The main registering body for psychotherapists is the United Kingdom Council for Psychotherapy (UKCP; www.psychotherapy.org.uk).

Cognitive behavioural therapy

CBT is a talking therapy that helps children to make sense of problems. It gives children a way of talking about how they think about themselves and their lives, and helps them understand how what they do affects their thoughts and feelings. It can help change how people think (cognitive) and what they do (behaviour). CBT is unusual among talking therapies because it focuses on the here and now rather than looking for causes for problems in the past. Contact the British Association for Behavioural and Cognitive Psychotherapies for more information (www.babcp.com).

Of course, talking therapies are not for everyone, and a lot of children with ADHD, particularly older boys, may not be all that responsive.

> 66 *These kids really don't want to sit and talk about their problems to anybody, so those types of therapy don't work for them. A lot of other kids love to talk about their conditions and what is happening to them, and how it affects them, in fact you can't shut them up, but generally the kids with ADHD don't like to talk about things and frankly don't have the concentration, focus or interest to do it.* 99
> **Billy's mum, who runs an ADHD support group**

> ## Why Try?
> Some parents of teenagers found the Why Try? programme helpful. This is a multi-sensory CBT programme designed to build critical social and emotional skills in children using hip-hop music and activities to address many of the skills they lack. It tackles anger management, low self-esteem, encourages youngsters to get out of gangs, helping them to be more resilient, to understand the mistakes they keep making and how they get stuck in a rut with recurring problems so they never move forward. Very significant for ADHD, the programme helps them to understand how the decisions they make have consequences and to work out how to set goals. Originally developed in America, the programme has been brought into a lot of schools around the UK. It is a postcode lottery whether it is available near you, but you can find out more at the ADDISS website (www.addiss.co.uk).

Behaviour therapy

This concentrates on the actual behaviour of the child, at home or at school, to find ways of changing or improving problematic behaviour so that the child feels better able to deal with situations they find difficult, to learn at school and to get on with other people. Behaviour therapists analyse the details of what a child does in different situations and come up with a plan for the individual child and also for the parents and carers, finding ways to encourage and reward positive behaviour.

Family therapy

Family therapy puts a lot of significance on what happens within the family and family therapists work with members of the family together to help the child.

66 *Parent training, behavioural work and cognitive behavioural work can help the child before medication needs to be considered, but if he doesn't respond*

*enough to that kind of help – which should always
be tried first – then it becomes sensible to try Ritalin
as well.* **"**
*Professor Tim Kendall, Director of the National
Collaborative Centre for Mental Health, who helped to
formulate the NICE guideline on ADHD*

The medication minefield

You will probably have noticed that from time to time the issue
of ADHD explodes into the media, usually as part of a controversy
about whether it is appropriate to medicate it in the way that we
do (and usually associated with the drug Ritalin). But as you'll see
in this chapter, many parents have found medication invaluable
in helping their child, and we'll also hear from children who have
used it too. However, some feel that the use of medication is too
readily sought.

" *There has been a gradual increase over the last
15 years in the use of Ritalin. There is good evidence
that Ritalin has good effects on performance in school
and the ability to make friends. Ritalin is amphetamine-
like, but, though there are similarities in its chemical
structure, it is not an amphetamine derivative. There
are concerns that people can be put off seeking
treatment for their children with ADHD as there has
been so much controversy and focus on Ritalin.* **"**
Professor Tim Kendall

The decision to start your child on medication mustn't be
taken lightly – and we'll take you through the pros and cons of
medication, to ensure you have the information you need.

How does it work?

ADHD medications usually cause a short-lived improvement after
each dose is taken, not a permanent cure. They give a window for

someone with ADHD to feel calmer, concentrate better, be less impulsive and learn better.

These are 'controlled' drugs, so their availability and use is monitored more closely than other prescription medicines. Your child will probably be given small dosages at first which will be increased gradually if necessary. Regular check-ups by your GP will help monitor side-effects and check that the treatment continues to be effective. If your child seems to have improved and is stable, the GP may well recommend a break in treatment, perhaps over a weekend or in the school holidays, which will give an indication of how well they can manage without it.

Three types of medication are used for ADHD in the UK.

1. Methylphenidate (Ritalin) is one of the most commonly used medications for ADHD in the UK. It is known as a central nervous system stimulant and is thought to stimulate a part of the brain that changes mental and behavioural reactions. It can be used under medical supervision by children over six years old and by teenagers, either as immediate-release tablets (small doses two or three times a day), or as modified-release tablets taken once a day, usually in the morning (this slow release medication is called Concerta). These tablets are stronger, which can be a disadvantage, but are more convenient as children do not then have to take doses in school. The children are regularly monitored for harmful side-effects, such as increase in blood pressure, trouble sleeping, headaches and mood swings. Some, such as loss of appetite can be eased by taking the medication with a meal or snack. Teenagers should avoid alcohol during treatment as it can make side-effects more severe.
2. Dexamfetamine works in the same way as methylphenidate, and can be particularly effective in controlling hyperactivity. It is usually taken as a daily tablet, and your child will be monitored for the same side-effects as those of methylphenidate.
3. Atomoxetine increases the amount of the brain chemical noradrenaline which passes messages between brain cells, so

aiding concentration and helping to control impulses. Like the others it must be monitored by your GP and specialist; there is a note of caution here in that some studies have shown that a small proportion of those who take the drug may have suicidal thoughts. Other side-effects can include nausea, waking early, irritability and dizziness.

Parents whose children have used medication, which is usually Ritalin or the slow-release Concerta in the first instance, report that it often has an almost instant effect, as it isn't a drug that takes a while to get into the system. It generally works itself out of the system on the same day it is taken, meaning that if the child doesn't take it the next day he will go back to what is normal for him.

> 66 *I found that the one that worked the best was the Concerta, slow-release Ritalin. With the other version you get very up and down periods and you end up having to try and give it at the right time for the best effect, and it all becomes very complicated. So when they introduced the slow-release version it had a profound effect. It ironed out the ups and downs, which was great.* 99
> **Sylvie, whose son, Ed, was diagnosed with ADHD and autism at three years old**

Pros and cons of medication

When a medication is being prescribed for your child you should check with the specialist what they feel about any other conditions your child may have, the side-effects and how they may affect him, the dosage times, and how they may impact on the schoolday.

Medication clearly has a place in treatment, and there is no doubt that it can be helpful; but there are always many factors that must be considered, and there can be significant side-effects.

66 *When we saw the doctor she was trying to explain
to Charlie how he might feel when he took the
medicine and about the side-effects and I had to
quietly ask her to stop. I explained that he is the kind of
child that if you tell him about the side-effects he might
have then he will have every single one of them.* 99
Charlie's mum

Studies show that children who take medication for their ADHD
experience both positive and negative effects. Many of the children
surveyed in a recent study on attitudes to ADHD medication,
carried out by researchers at the London School of Economics,
felt that medication helped to control their hyperactivity and
behaviour, increased their concentration and meant that they got
better marks for school work. They did not necessarily like being
on medication, but they were willing to put up with the 'annoying'
aspects of taking it in return for what they saw as benefits.

The main benefit the children saw was in helping their social
behaviour, making them less disruptive and, consequently,
improving their relationships with friends, rather than in
improving their school work.

A lot of them had side-effects such as sleep problems and reduced
appetite, stomach aches and headaches, and some also disliked
the taste of the medicine, but these things didn't seem to bother
them over-much. Some worried about feeling less sociable, with a
sense of not being their usual selves.

66 *He has been on medicine for four weeks and his
teacher says she is starting to notice a difference. My
main concern about the medication was that he has
a lively, bubbly personality, very likeable and very soft
and loving though he can turn at the flick of a switch.
I was worried in case the medication would knock all
that out of him. Another worry is that he is a tall, skinny
boy and the medication is affecting his appetite. We
are having to coax him to eat a bit, which is new. He*

has to eat before his medication and we know they will
keep an eye on him and weigh him and measure his
blood pressure. 99
Joan, Charlie's grandmother

All the children interviewed felt they needed to be on their tablets; older ones were more likely to be looking ahead to a time when they could manage without them. They believed that medication was the most effective available treatment for their ADHD symptoms, but they understood that even with the diagnosis of ADHD and effective drug treatment they still had responsibility for their own behaviour.

Interviewees did not want others to know about their taking medication because they were worried about being laughed at. A number also said that they felt embarrassed about having to leave the classroom to be given their medication.

The thing the group expressed really strongly was a wish for better understanding of ADHD by the public and by their teachers. They felt this would create empathy and relieve them of some of the stigma attached to a diagnosis of ADHD.

66 *The first week he was taking his tablets he bit a*
child at school, which he has never done at all. I asked
him why he had done it, and he said that someone had
told him the reason he had the medicine was that his
brain didn't tell his body what to do properly, so he
didn't know what he was doing. For him to come out
with that, he had obviously had the idea put in his head
by the adult who had told him what they thought about
the medicine. So I had to be very firm with him that he
does know what he is doing and he must not use that
as an excuse, he is responsible for himself and what he
does. He knows that really, he has had it drummed into
him, and I wish that people at school would just think
before they speak. 99
Charlie's mum

What children see as the pros and cons of medication

Pros

Some children feel the medication:

- helps control behaviour and therefore improves relationships with friends
- makes it easier to concentrate on schoolwork and get better marks
- enables them to concentrate on quiet activities like computer games
- makes them calmer.

Cons

Others feel the medication:

- takes away their personality
- affects their appetite, and causes a stomach ache
- can have a bad effect on sleeping
- can be awkward and embarrassing to take in school
- can have a nasty taste.

> 66 *There were both good and bad things about the medication. For instance, when he went for his tennis lesson for the first time after his prescription, the coach said that it was amazing that for the first time he was listening to what he was told, but that his reactions were off, so he couldn't play as well as usual. He couldn't react fast enough to the ball.* 99
> **Ben's mum**

> 66 *Since he has been taking the medication he is sometimes a bit quiet and withdrawn – not dopey or drowsy, I wouldn't want him to take it if it was having that kind of effect – but more as if he wants to be in his own little world. Whereas normally in the past he was just charging around, now he wants to sit and play on the computer. He is just taking himself off to do*

something quiet, the way the other children do, but it is really weird to see him be like that. 💬
Charlie's mum

The effect of Ritalin on growth

💬 *We know that Ritalin affects growth, and we are talking about children with growing brains so we should not use it continuously. If you stop the treatment, say for the school summer holidays, then growth will catch up.*

It interferes with growth because it inhibits appetite in the day and leads to ravenous hunger in the evening – which is not good. It appears to inhibit the production of growth hormone also, so it has two ways of interfering with metabolic function. We are also not sure of the effect on growing brains yet. 💬
Professor Tim Kendall

💬 *The reason that we have given the Ritalin up is that it really, really has knocked Patrick's sleep in the sense of his being completely unable to get to sleep. He would still be awake at 11 or 12 at night, and he has to travel a long way to his school so needs to be up at 6.30am. We just felt it couldn't be right for an 11-year-old to be getting about six hours' sleep.* 💬
Patrick's mum

What parents think about medication

You won't be surprised to discover that there are a lot of different views about medication. After all, each child is an individual, and they are affected in different ways both by the condition and the medication for it. Health professionals have their own opinions, but for the low-down on real-life experience you have to go back to the parents.

66 When Sally got her first dose of Ritalin within 10 minutes she sat down and calmed down. She just relaxed, which hadn't happened before. She never talked about it or how it made her feel, never admitted it helped or that she liked it. In her mind, she would rather not have had to take it, because she didn't like being different. 99

Sally's mum

66 Ben doesn't like Ritalin, but the difference when he was taking it was phenomenal. Because he is so articulate he could explain his feelings about being on Ritalin quite well. He said he felt like it took away all his electricity. His doctor explained it quite well to us in terms of – if everyone else goes out to a party and has a few drinks they get really buzzy and high; and they have a great time and then they go home and go to sleep. And when they wake up the next morning they feel normal. Kids with ADHD are in that party mode all the time – that is how they live day to day. When they take Ritalin that is how they come back to normal, but they don't like being normal because it is not what they are used to. 99

Ben's mum

66 Billy had already been in the pupil referral unit and we had been running backwards and forwards to school three or four times a day because he was on the verge of expulsion. After three weeks of taking the medication he just blended into the background and his teachers were astonished at the transformation in him. I know a lot of parents have different views on the medication but for us, when he started taking it in his final year at school he went from a kid who was about to be expelled to a kid who walked out with six GCSE passes. My heart breaks for what he could have achieved if we could have sorted it out and got him on the medication sooner. 99

Billy's mum

66 The first couple of days he was withdrawn and didn't seem like himself. But I think he was just obviously finding that it was making his brain tick in a different way, and I don't think he could understand why he was feeling a bit different. But now he is just getting on with it and I think it is really positive. 99
Charlie's mum

66 A lot of people seem to be anti-drugs, for us Ritalin was the thing that enabled our son to go to secondary school and concentrate and learn. I'm not sure that he would have had the ability to tackle any GCSEs without it. 99
Ed's mum

66 I feel that the combination of help from an educational psychologist, the carefully controlled and limited prescription of Ritalin and sessions with a counsellor have been so effective that they have been worth everything they cost in terms of getting things sorted out and making him happy, confident and on track for the future. He is not sure whether to continue Ritalin for university but it helps so much with concentration that he is keen to take it in term time. 99
Hugh's mum

66 I wouldn't have noticed it particularly, as far as home life was concerned – certainly I didn't see any of that miraculous thing that appears on TV documentaries where 20 minutes after a child has had Ritalin they calm down. I didn't feel that that was the case for us at all. In fact it was quite difficult to feel that Saturday and Sunday were any different to the way that they were pre-Ritalin. I maybe feel that it gave him a bit more time to think before he acted, but at school they were saying great things about it. 99
Patrick's mum

66 *When the medication works it works really well. When you have a proper, careful diagnosis, monitoring the medication can transform a child's life. Both my children have been on medication and I know what it has done for them. My older boy has a degree in maths and runs his own business, and he says that if it hadn't been for the medication he would be sleeping on the streets.* 99

Andrea Bilbow, mother of two sons with ADHD and founder of the ADHD support group and charity ADDISS

The decision to use medication isn't an easy one, and you have to balance up the pros and the cons for your child. But the dosage can be controlled, and dosage and effects will always be carefully monitored by your specialist and your GP.

Other treatments and therapies recommended by parents

As well as the treatments listed in this chapter, there are other treatments that the parents we interviewed for this book found useful. It is worth having a look to see if you feel that some of them might be worth a try. Some have to be paid for, others are free.

Relaxation

Relaxation techniques such as deep breathing can be very beneficial for ADHD sufferers. There is a recommendation to combine them with the use of positive imagery – such as the child imagining doing well in the classroom, which might lead to a real-life improvement once the child has allowed for the possibility. You could get a relaxation tape, and listen to it together, or if you find a relaxation class in your area it might do you both a power of good. Massage can be very beneficial to tense and anxious children and several parents report long-term good effects from regular massages.

Cranial osteopathy is a gentle, non-invasive treatment, which gets an enthusiastic thumbs up from quite a few parents. The Osteopathic Centre for Children, a charitable organisation specialising in paediatric osteopathy, treats many children with ADHD. To find your nearest source of treatment visit www.occ.uk.com or call 020 8875 5290.

Focusing on skills

There is a school of thought that acquiring new skills such as juggling or chess helps make new connections in the brain, and some parents also recommend memory and sequencing exercises that can be played as games. One example is the coin game, where you arrange five different coins in a pattern, then mix them up and repeat the exact pattern with a timer. When the time taken improves, make a more difficult pattern.

In much the same way, doing picture puzzles or crosswords can improve attention and concentration. It is lovely for a child if you sit down with him and either share his puzzle or do one of your own.

Piano lessons can be very enjoyable, and have benefits for concentration and control. Other parents have found the benefits of music therapy as an adjunct to other treatments. This therapy is not the same as music lessons, as the child does not learn to play an instrument, though they may gain some musical skills. Find out more at www.nordoff-robbins.org.uk (020 7267 4496) or find a therapist in your area via the British Association for Music Therapy (www.bamt.org; 020 7837 6100).

Auditory integration training (AIT)

Some parents have found AIT effective as a means to reduce some ADHD symptoms. AIT uses filtered and modulated frequencies embedded into music listened to through headphones to help retrain a disorganised auditory system. This is thought to help normalise the senses so that improvements are seen in focus, attention and ability to concentrate even in noisy environments. Visit www.auditoryintegration.net for more details.

Throughout the rest of the book we'll be looking at other ways of helping your child – from your parenting technique and style, to the food he eats. Together with the treatments and therapies listed in this chapter, you can help your child as he tries to deal with his ADHD.

4

Practical parenting
How you can help

If you are reading this book, you are clearly a parent who wants to make things better for your child. You may have struggled with the feeling that you are being judged for poor parenting and your child's bad behaviour by friends, other parents and healthcare professionals alike.

But as we mentioned in Chapter 1, there are many causes of ADHD. Your parenting style will not have caused ADHD, but the way you parent can certainly help your child live with the condition, and can help the rest of your family, too.

> 66 *ADHD can manifest itself from a very young age. We need to find ways to help parents as early as possible, from the stage of children aged three or younger, long before we could prescribe any medication, which is at age six at the youngest. Teaching useful parenting tactics at an early stage can in many cases prevent the need for medication later on.* 99
> *Professor Tim Kendall*

Parenting skills

It can seem daunting to try to modify the behaviour of a child whose very nature seems to be difficult and extremely energetic. It is probably futile, even damaging, to try to force him to be like everybody else his age. However, with the right approach you may be able to modify destructive behaviour patterns and help your child find some self-belief to counter the negativity and lack of confidence that are among the long-term effects of ADHD.

It is true to say that many parents think they could improve their parenting skills. Most of us benefit from impartial advice and support with the thorny problems of bringing up children, and this is especially the case with something as demanding as ADHD.

Evidence suggests that if parents get help dealing with their child's behaviour early enough the chance of a formal diagnosis decreases. The younger your child is when you start the better. If you start with a nursery school-age child you can increase the chances of successful treatment, and decrease the chances of your child exhibiting problem behaviour at school.

> 66 It is important to say that every parent has difficulty as their child grows up. That is not to say that problems such as ADHD are caused by parenting, rather that they can often be made a lot better by informed parenting, and in this context parenting classes can help to broaden our perspective. 99
> **Professor Tim Kendall**

Children with ADHD tend to be much more prone to behavioural problems because they don't stop and think. They have a partial attention span so if you say 'Don't jump in the puddle' they will hear 'Jump in the puddle' and that is exactly what they will do. So the usual parenting mechanisms often don't work and you will need some pretty rigid rules (see below).

Some basic rules for parents

- **Have clear rules and clear boundaries**. Make sure that there are clear, pre-agreed consequences for breaking rules, and for unacceptable behaviour, and enforce them. Write and hang them up in a place where the children can easily read them.
- **Be consistent and firm**. Once you have established your ground rules, be consistent in rewarding good behaviour and discouraging bad behaviour. Remember that a child with ADHD finds it very hard to adapt to change, so keep things as ordered and consistent as possible
- **Minimise the negatives**. Part of the deal has to be that parents don't lose their tempers, flare up and say inappropriate things. You need to try to stay calm, apply these consequences as agreed and move on from the situation.
- **Be warm and loving**. While it's key to be consistent and follow any consequences through, remember to tell your child that you love him, and show him affection and warmth.
- **Praise the good behaviour**. We are all wonderful at noticing bad behaviour immediately and giving children our undivided attention when they do bad things, but we are not so good at noticing good behaviour and giving them undivided attention for that. We have to get better at that too. (See below.)
- **Pick your battles**. You have to work out which aspects of your child's behaviour you personally find intolerable, such as fighting with other children or verbal abuse. Then work out the things that bother you the least, and be prepared to put up with them – indefinitely if necessary. Let some things go, and be prepared to compromise.

> ❝ I saw an article recently by someone who just wanted to be controversial, which said ADHD doesn't really exist. It is just bad parenting and that made me so angry. Actually I think all the good stuff – the fact that I can concentrate to a certain extent – is just from being made to as a kid, and that is down to mum. In the long run it is incredibly damaging if you are allowed to use something like a label of ADHD as an excuse

for everything and a reason not to do things. You need some rigidity from your parents and teachers. **99**
Hugh

> **TIP** In Chapter 5 we'll look at tactics you can use on a day-to-day basis to make your home and family life easier, including introducing a routine to help your child.

Praise and rewards

Organised systems of rewards and consequences are very helpful for ADHD children. Explain clearly what happens when the rules are obeyed, and what happens when they are broken. Stick with the system and follow through consistently with a reward or a consequence.

A child with ADHD gets so much criticism at school and in the larger world that every bit of praise matters even more to him, as it may not come his way very often. So, try never to miss an opportunity for praise and encouragement, no matter how small the achievement, even if it is something that you would take for granted in another child.

- Reward with praise, activities or a privilege rather than with food or toys. For instance, if he manages a trip to the supermarket he might get some computer time, or a game with you. Get him to help decide what the rewards should be.
- Make the praise specific – 'You tidied up very well' – so he knows exactly what he has done right.
- Change the rewards fairly regularly, as children with ADHD will get bored if the reward is always the same.
- Younger children may like a star chart giving them a visual reminder of past successes.
- An immediate reward is much better than the promise of something in the future for ADHD children, but you might have success with small rewards that accumulate to lead to a big one.

- If a reward has been agreed as the consequence for some particular behaviour, always honour it. A child with ADHD responds to disappointment with greater frustration than his non-ADHD counterparts and things are likely to get noisy. Remember if he responds in this way that it is part of his character, and not something that he can easily control.
- In the case of bad behaviour, the consequences should have been established in advance, and should occur immediately after the misbehaviour so that there is no doubt about what has caused them.
- Removal of privileges can be an effective punishment.
- It is only fair to remove your child from situations or surroundings that trigger bad behaviour – for instance, the supermarket. If you see the signs of an impending melt-down try to intervene quickly and take him away or distract him. Often a child will suddenly explode with rage for no apparent reason. If this happens in public the best thing you can do is leave, with your child, as quickly and calmly as possible.
- After bad behaviour, when things have calmed down, ask him what he thinks he should have done instead.
- Toddlers with ADHD may show a lot of physical aggression and impulsivity. It is worth trying to teach them to channel this verbally – although you may have to put up with some cross and shouty language.
- 'Time-out', where you remove a child immediately (and without showing any emotion) from a situation that is threatening to be out of control, is a way for both you and the child to cool down. The child should be encouraged to see it as a valuable way of cooling down and getting some perspective on his behaviour, and should know that time-out will be an inevitable consequence of that kind of behaviour.

Parenting classes

If you sometimes feel a bit overwhelmed by the problems of being a parent, you are far from alone. You may also find that a lot of the parenting techniques that will help you to manage an ADHD child are not intuitive, and, as well as putting in place some of the suggestions here, it may help you to go on a parenting class or course.

All parents can benefit from a bit of outside wisdom from time to time, even if it is not always easy to admit it. Of course, the problems you face are not exactly the same as others, but in a lot of areas, such as sleeplessness, tantrums and general issues of behaviour, they are heightened versions of fairly universal issues.

So, while classes tailored specifically to the needs of parents of children with ADHD are not always easy to find, there are plenty of other parenting classes and courses that can be of help.

> 66 *Group support coupled with formal help can make a real difference. If you get parents together who have difficulties in common they can learn from each other's experience. This is the same approach as group therapy and can be very successful.* 99
> **Professor Tim Kendall**

> 66 *Some research from America showed that the children of parents who attend support groups do better than the children of parents who don't. ADHD is a condition where you can feel isolated. People don't understand and the media are always attacking the parents of children with ADHD. Belonging to a support group can be comforting and helpful; it is where you pick up tips. In a group you get support and feedback from other parents in the same boat. It is good to share.* 99
> **Andrea Bilbow**

Parenting classes give advice and information on bringing up children, and deal with how to handle behavioural problems and discipline. Here you are sure to find ideas and strategies that will help you, and that you may not have thought of before. Positive discipline and reflective listening are two skills that are important to learn, and may help to give you some new ideas and insights into why children behave the way they do.

You will be given tips about how to manage any stress and anger you are feeling yourself, and you may find these really useful. These classes also give you the chance to meet other parents and think not only about how you are bringing up your children, but also about how you were brought up yourself.

Evidence shows that positive and authoritative parenting, which uses love, respect, consistency, clear communication and empathy in the way you behave with your child has massive benefits for both sides. These skills are great for any parent to learn, but are even more important for parents of children with ADHD – your patience will be tested to the extreme, and your child will need clear, fair discipline.

How to find a class

To find a class, go through your GP surgery or social services, which can direct you to local authority-run schemes in your area, or contact Parentline Plus (www.familylives.org.uk; 0808 800 2222). These courses are free to parents and would generally run for two hours a week for six weeks. They cover specific areas and issues, such as understanding your child, harmony in the home or dealing with tantrums. There are also some classes that you can access privately.

The government website www.directgov.uk is another good place to start, as the website will direct you towards your local services and your nearest local authority children's centres, where a lot of courses are based.

For other sources of help and details of classes nationwide, visit www.parentinguk.org.

Barnardo's (www.barnardos.org.uk/adhdservices) runs a programme called 'The Parent Factor in ADHD', part of a range of services for families of children with ADHD and professionals dealing with them. The services aim to provide support that will help children and young people with ADHD to fulfil their potential. The parent programme is mainly available in the north-east of England and parts of Scotland, and it is hoped that it will become more widely available around the UK. Contact Barnado's North East for details. Feedback suggests that parents find the practical strategies, learning from others and reassurance offered in the programme beneficial. Some parents find that a lot of the content is common sense, but that being given the explanation that children are not behaving that way on purpose, that it is something in the make up of their brain and it is not their fault can help to put things in perspective.

1-2-3 Magic is a behavioural management programme designed by clinical psychologist Thomas Phelan. It is based around a simple-to-use counting method and is a tried and tested method of getting children to stop unwanted behaviours and encourage good ones. Specifically designed for the symptoms of ADHD, it is licensed in this country by the charity ADDISS. The parenting classes give you tactics to use to encourage positive behaviour. The third part of the programme is building self-esteem and encouraging family relationships. It can be delivered from the age of two to up to the age of 12, but with the maturity lag of some of these children you could use it until they were a bit older. There is also a second stage, 'Surviving Adolescence.' Parents can go on a programme which they can access through the NHS locally, or buy the book and DVD and teach themselves. This programme helps parents understand and manage the behaviours. For details, visit www.addiss.org.uk.

> ❝ 1-2-3 Magic saved my sanity. It is a totally different approach to normal parenting programmes. It is a quick way for worn-down parents to get to the root of the problem and manage the behaviour first. You can't have a positive relationship with your child if things have got to the stage where you are always screaming and shouting and getting really upset. The programme teaches parents first to tackle the behaviour and sort it out. If your child was having a tantrum in the supermarket this gives you a way of stopping it. Basically you are training your child to do what you want them to do and showing them that you are in charge. It teaches the parents to control their

own emotions as well so that they don't lose the plot.
One interesting feedback we have had is that, as a lot
of these parents have ADHD themselves, by doing
the course to help their children, they have learned to
control their own behaviour. 99
Andrea Bilbow

It is clear that parenting classes are a great way to acquire some extra parenting skills, and are suggested by NICE as a way to deal with ADHD. Sometimes they may give you all you need to sort out the problems, but it is unrealistic to expect that this will always be the case.

66 *Usually good parenting will prevent the*
complications of ADHD and it might help the parent
and the child to get on a bit better and understand
each other a bit better, but it will not cure ADHD.
In a severe case, I don't think anything will replace
medication, and that is not a cure. 99
Dr Dinah Jayson

Ways to help yourself

Being the parent of a child with ADHD is at best tiring, and worst, extremely stressful. You are an important source of strength and order for your child, so if you get overtired or run out of patience the whole structure is rocked. Set the good example of eating healthily, taking exercise and getting plenty of sleep, and find ways of reducing stress, even if it is just a soak in the bath at night. Ensuring you are coping will directly benefit your child – you'll have more energy to give him. Here are some tips how other parents have coped and managed their own emotions.

- Stay as calm as you can, even in the face of horrible behaviour. Remember your child cannot help it and it is not really directed at you. If your child is getting into a state, try to change the scene by getting him out into the garden or some other safe place.

- If you do feel that you are starting to lose your temper with your child hand over to someone else for a few minutes if you can. If you are on your own, and you feel it is safe, say that you are going to the bathroom and have 10 minutes to cool off a bit and clear your head.
- Hang on to the perspective that your child's behaviour is related to a disorder and is generally not intentional.
- If friends or family members offer to help out with some babysitting, accept – but leave them with a clear idea of what may crop up, and what the house rules are.
- Be prepared to compromise – if your child has completed one task but not managed another it may be best to let the second thing go and praise the first. Keep your expectations realistic.
- Pinpoint regular conflict/trigger points such as the supermarket, and either avoid them or work out a clear strategy for dealing with them.
- If you do get ill or feel like you really aren't coping, acknowledge it, and get some help.

> ❝ I went for some therapy myself, and as she heard the dramas of our life with Ben unfold each week the therapist eventually said, 'I actually think you would be mad not to be depressed by all of this.' It has affected my life to a huge degree. ❞
> **Ben's mum**

Focusing on the positives

Granted, this may be a big ask on the most difficult days when your child has been tearing around the house at 100 miles an hour, but the energy, enthusiasm and creativity displayed by many children with ADHD can be a rewarding part of the condition if you can encourage them. The comedian Rory Bremner, by his own diagnosis a lifelong ADHD sufferer, can see many advantages: 'I like the way I am – lots of plates spinning at once – in a way it is more like an attention surfeit than an attention deficit, our minds work faster and make quicker connections.'

66 *Hugh is very good at talking to people and he can talk his way in anywhere and talk to anyone, and he is very astute at working people out. Maybe the extreme chattiness is part of the general hyperness of the condition.* 99
Hugh's mum

A family's story

Daisy is 12 and had ADHD and other learning difficulties diagnosed when she was five. Her mother Laura is a GP, and she suspects that she has the condition herself and can also see the signs of it in Daisy's younger brother:

Five is young by some standards, and Daisy has pretty much been on medication since then. It has helped enormously. When we started on it my husband (also a GP) was not at all keen, so we started with a small dose on school mornings to see what happened. The teacher was a bit pale and horrified when we told her, but it made a massive difference. I would say it just makes a difference to Daisy's focus and concentration; it has never subdued her. The only problem we have with it is that it does affect her sleep because of nightmares, which does seem cruel.

She was on a small dose for a while and the school could not believe the difference it made. Then we saw a consultant a year later and he said that she was on a piddly dose, and what is more for the sake of family sanity we should use it at home. That completely transformed our family life. She has a younger brother who is 10. I am pretty certain he has ADHD too, but no one wants to know that. He is incredibly fidgety, he has a zero concentration span and he is really hyperactive all over the place. His father doesn't want to go down that route with his son. The trouble is he is in a school where he is bumping along at the bottom in a major way and they just can't make sense of it. He doesn't concentrate, they say, he has to get up and wander around all the time. It is so clear to me that ADHD is his problem, but I am a lone voice. He has problems with friendships. He is a very likeable little fellow, and he has lots of friends, but no real close mates.

We have seen three lots of educational psychologists, and they can't make any sense of him at all. I think he has some kind of learning issue as well. He can't tell the time, his reading and writing are gradually getting there but he is way behind his peers. He has no short-term memory. You can tell him something and then you go back to it and it is as if he has never done it before. To me that is a function of having no attention span. He was not concentrating first time round so he has never processed the information. He has been in two schools and never have they been very proactive about it. I really want him to be assessed, even if we don't go down the medication route. That window for learning for children is really narrow, and I feel so passionately that we could miss the boat. It absolutely turned my daughter around so much, that I wish he could have a trial of the medication.

As a parent you are so desperate for some help and some support, and some way to make sense of it all, and as things are at the moment, a lot of what help is available comes too late for most families.

We were perhaps unusual in getting Daisy diagnosed quite young. I feel very passionately that we should be having much more intervention very early on because I knew, as did my husband, that my poor little scrap really had problems from the start. All parents know when something is not right with their child and the system is very good at placating and temporising and giving false reassurance. What happens is that families struggle and struggle and when they do re-present it is quite late and a lot more could have been done for the child, and the parents could have had more help. The statementing process takes so much time, and then there are often appeals when it goes wrong and all that leads to so much wasted energy and emotion.

With our daughter we knew within months that something was amiss. She was very unrewarding. I didn't get any of the feedback from her that I got when my son arrived. She also has developmental dyspraxia – and it is very difficult to pick the

continued

continued from previous page

conditions apart because all these things are different bits of spectra. You could look at my daughter from a dyspraxia point of view and say it is all down to that or you could look at her from an ADHD point of view and say it is all that. She has big processing issues and problems with communications skills. She can't get across what she wants to tell you in the way that most people would – it all comes out a bit upside down and inside out, a bit jumbly hopeless. So from a very young age she was unrewarding and unresponsive – she didn't turn her head so we actually thought she had a hearing issue to start with and this was at six months so we pursued that. A bit more time went by and that seemed to be a bit better, and she was growing and developing and some things seemed to be improving, though she was always behind the normal.

We had her in a lovely nursery when she was three and we were planning to go abroad for a while, at which point the headmistress took me to one side and said to me that they had real concerns about Daisy. They probably wouldn't have mentioned anything to us at that stage if we hadn't been going away. She didn't want me to take her to another nursery and for them to say 'Don't you realise your child has got real problems?' She said that they wouldn't have done anything about the problems yet because children are all so different in the way they develop and normally they would just wait and see, but she thought she ought to tell me. I broke down because I was so relieved to know that it wasn't just me, that there really was something that wasn't right. When we got back to the UK, we went through an extensive assessment process with Daisy, but I had to suggest to the consultant that I thought she might have ADHD. As a professional parent I seem to have driven so much of this myself.

I am almost at the point of getting hold of the NICE guidelines with a marker pen and marking up all the things that we have never been offered, and that we have no prospect of being offered. Even as a health professional myself I cannot make the system work for us.

5

Home life and how to make it work

By putting together a selection of strategies and routines that work for you both, dealing with your child will become much easier. You have to remember that his ADHD is as frustrating for him as it is for you. Displays of the behaviour may drive you crazy – but remember that your child probably wants to sit quietly, or be organised and tidy and do what he is told – he just can't do it.

He often has problems with thinking ahead, finishing tasks, getting organised or controlling impulsive actions. You have to take some of this on for him, so that over time the example you set may rub off and he may gradually do it for himself, and this is one of the reasons that the sooner you start the better for your child.

Your child may exhaust you with behaviour that is fearless, impulsive and generally chaotic, but hold fast to the knowledge that as a parent there is a lot you can do to help. A positive attitude and common sense will help the whole family.

> 66 *I find that many conditions can be made easier to cope with by using the same basic tactics. Children respond well to structure – and you have to be very fair, but firm. Stay calm. Tell them when their behaviour is unacceptable. If they know they can go over a boundary, they will. I keep the boundaries the same, so the girl I look after knows where she is, and this is the same for all children with special needs. Structure is all-important. Activity, Boundaries, Continuity are my ABC for dealing with ADHD.* 99
> **Jackie, who has worked with children with special needs for many years, and currently helps a 12-year-old girl with ADHD**

Tactics that work with ADHD children

Structure and routine

It is more likely that an ADHD child will be able to succeed with a task when it is something predictable and happening in a place where he expects it to. A child with ADHD acts on his impulses, he just can't help it, and he never thinks about cause and effect. As much as you can, you need to do it for him, keep talking about how one thing leads to another, and hope that, over time, he will start to understand. Here are some tips on how to bring in structure to his life.

- Establish a routine, and stick to it as much as you can. If there is a time and a place for everything in his everyday life that will help him to understand what is expected of him and do it.
- Have simple routines and timings that go with meals, homework, play and bed, broken down into easy steps if necessary.
- Consider using a timer to mark out homework time, play time, getting ready for bed time as a way of reinforcing the schedule.

- Issues of tidiness and organisation are often a big problem for these children and you can help a lot by things such as labelling drawers, so things are easy to find. Otherwise, you may find him going through the lot and causing chaos just to track down one thing. Keep his environment tidy and organised, and that may help him to pick up on some of these qualities for himself.
- Help your child to lay out his clothes for tomorrow before going to bed to save stress in the morning. Make sure he has everything he needs for school in a set place, where he will be sure to pick it up in the morning.
- If you are asking him to do something, be very specific. Instead of asking him to tidy up, for instance, ask him to put the toys in the toybox and the cups in the kitchen. Then give him specific praise when he gets it right.

> 66 Thinking back to things that might have been pointers to the ADHD – Hugh was always spectacularly untidy. I used to beg him to put things in the same place every night so that he could find them in the morning, but he just couldn't do it. Now he does, but it has been a long struggle. 99
> Hugh's mum

> 66 One thing that we have noticed is crucial for Charlie is routines. He has to know what is happening when. His mum prepared him for his medication for a couple of weeks beforehand so he had a chance to get used to the idea and didn't feel he was having anything sprung on him. We have always noticed that he can cope much better if he knows what is going to happen in advance. 99
> Charlie's grandmother

Break down tasks to aid concentration

When asking your child to do something, bear in mind that his brain works differently, and he will need more structure than usual. Here are some top tips to help him.

- Break down tasks into small steps and one at a time – ADHD children often have problems with planning, sequencing and organising.
- Make frequent checks on the child – he needs much more scaffolding to keep him on task.
- Get him to repeat back to you whatever you have said so that you can be sure that he has heard it.
- Give him something to reward completion of a task straight away because he cannot cope with delayed gratification. Maybe have a delayed reward as well, but if he doesn't get something right in front of him he just loses interest.

When parenting a child with ADHD it's crucial to make sure your behaviour does not echo your child's. This can be very hard if you've got ADHD yourself when it is important to find self-calming mechanisms to calm down, walk away and prevent the eruptions happening.

Keep him busy and active – but not too busy

Simplify the schedule. It is important to be active but this does not have to involve a constant round of after-school activities. Some ADHD children thrive on this, but you will soon be able to tell if your child is over-extended, because he will become over-tired, with consequent disastrous effects on behaviour.

- The ADHD child needs a lot of activity. Keep him doing something and when he is good remember to reward and praise him. He needs to know he has done something good.
- When you have all day with him, have the next activity lined up in your mind so you are one step ahead. Get the next thing ready so he doesn't get bored and frustrated. Time with nothing to do may make him act up, but try to keep him busy without him having so much to do that it becomes overwhelming. If that happens he may act up even more.

- Plan out everything that needs to be done in the day and break it down into manageable chunks for him. Then if you can, have times when he can choose to do something he enjoys as a reward for doing the stuff he has to do.
- Organise simple things to fill up the time like helping you cook, playing a board game or drawing. Try not to resort to the television or computer games too much, as if they are too exciting, your child's behaviour may respond.
- If he does what you have asked him, even if it is just clearing up a plate, then have a reward ready for him.
- Have a quiet place that he can go to if he needs to – and try to have somewhere separate that siblings can go to if it all gets too much.

The benefits of exercise

A child with ADHD often has bags of surplus energy. Organised sports can help him to use up some of his energy in healthy ways, and also help to focus his attention on skills and specific movements.

> ❝ With kids with ADHD, you can wear them down to the ground and they will still be spinning at 3am. We used to have lovely family holidays to places like America, but they were always really tiring for us because no matter how many activities we put in place we could never make Ben tired, and it was exhausting for us trying to contain him. With most kids you could wear them out physically with activity and they would go to sleep; with ADHD it can often make them more hyped up and make them worse. Ben would always have things like Game Boys on holiday but there would be a total panic if the batteries ran out, thinking of how we could contain him until we got some more. ❞
> **Ben's mum**

ADHD children seem to perform noticeably better when they are interested in something, so search out activities that hold your child's interest and concentration.

> ❝ Sally has lots of energy and it was great when that was harnessed into sport. The more sport she played the calmer she was, and she was very fit. She could be channelled into something like that with great enthusiasm, and in that way you can see the drive behind ADHD can be a positive. ❞
> **Sally's mum**

- Physical activity improves concentration, can lessen anxiety and depression and, importantly for ADHD children, can lead to better sleep.
- Swimming, tennis and other sports that focus the attention while limiting peripheral distractions are good options.
- Sign up for a sport that your child enjoys, and that suits his strengths. Sports that leave participants sitting on the sidelines for long periods of time, such as cricket, are not ideal. It may be better to stick with individual or team sports such as hockey or football that need constant motion. Do bear in mind that certain team sports require continual alertness, such as football or basketball, so they may not be ideal for a child with concentration issues.
- Yoga or tai kwon do, which emphasise mental control as they work on the body, can be highly beneficial for ADHD children.
- Use that surplus energy in a positive way – lots of running around at break time may help with focus in class; having something like a squeezy ball or putty to squeeze in his hands in lessons can help, too.
- Trampolining can work off lots of energy. If you have space, you could put a mini-trampoline in your back garden.

> ❝ In exams you are allowed toilet breaks. I noticed that when I got up and went out to the toilet in an exam it made my mind clearer. In Japanese offices, they have 10-minute breaks where the staff go up on the roof and do star jumps to get the blood flowing, I came up with the idea that if I went for two toilet breaks (three seems like taking the mick) and jogged

*on the spot really quickly, and did some star jumps
and then sprinted back to the exam room, it was really
energising. You may feel like an idiot but have enough
confidence to know that it will help you and you will
come back feeling better.* 🎗
Hugh

Eating and diet

Food can affect any child's mental state, and although it does
not appear that diet is a direct cause of ADHD, mental state can
always affect behaviour, which is obviously pretty crucial for
children with ADHD. Monitoring what your child eats, when and
how much can only be a help. All children will benefit from fresh,
wholesome foods and staying away from junk food as much as
possible.

Sugar

The advice on the NHS website states clearly that there is no
evidence that sugar causes the symptoms of ADHD, but eating a
lot of sweet foods and drinks is not the way to good nutrition, so
any sensible restrictions you make in this area will be generally
beneficial.

Additives

Some food colour additives are still implicated in some
hyperactivity, and advice from the British Nutrition Foundation
(www.bnf.org.uk) is to try to avoid some particular artificial
colour additives if your child shows signs of hyperactivity as they
have been linked to a negative effect on behaviour.

> TIP It is wise to avoid the following food colour additives:
> sunset yellow (E110), quinoline yellow (E104),
> carmoisine (E122), allura red (E129), tartrazine (E102) and
> ponceau 4R (E124). Check the ingredients of packaged food.

As well as avoiding additives, it does seem that keeping an eye on what your child eats, and modifying his diet in healthy directions can help the symptoms of ADHD. Regular mealtimes are good for everyone, and especially for ADHD sufferers, whose characteristic impulsiveness and distractedness can lead to missed meals, overeating and generally disordered eating. There is some evidence that meals and snacks taken at most three hours apart can be a help.

Caffeine

As you probably know from your own tea or coffee intake, caffeine is a stimulant. Giving an already hyperactive child more stimulation is not a good idea, and therefore you should look to exclude caffeine wherever possible.

Processed food

Apart from the avoidance of the additives mentioned above, there is no reason to avoid processed foods specifically for ADHD, but for general health it is good to have as much freshly prepared food as is possible.

Does it work?

The jury is still out on the significance of fish oil supplements or the exclusion of additives in the diet. However, while there are no hard and fast recommendations to go on, there is plenty of evidence from other parents that these things have played a helpful part in improving the effects of ADHD in their children. There can certainly be no harm in paying close attention to your child's diet and making it as healthy as possible.

> **TIP** One of the side-effects of medication can be that appetite decreases during the day and the child finds it hard to eat and then eats voraciously in the evening when the medication wears off. It is important to be aware of this.

Top tips for your child's diet

- Set a good example by adopting a healthy diet yourself.
- Make mealtimes regular and routine. Without help from his parents, the ADHD child may not eat for hours, then just shovel down whatever is around which can have disastrous consequences for him both physically and emotionally.
- Eating small meals more often may help your child with ADHD. Have regular meals and snack breaks no more than three hours apart. A regular intake of food makes sense for a group of children who, by definition, are using up a lot of energy, and mentally, mealtimes provide a necessary break and relaxation which is an important part of the routine of the day.
- Getting poor eaters to help you cook can spark their interest.
- If you think that your child becomes more hyperactive after eating certain foods it may be a good idea to keep a food diary and discuss your findings with your GP or a nutritionist.

> 66 We tried changing his diet and leaving out additives and preservatives and looking at all the E numbers and things but not to any avail. We did find that he was better not having fizzy drinks as he got older. He would want to be like everyone else and have coke, and we had to say no because we knew what the consequences would be. 99
> Charlie's grandmother

- Some parents report that omega-3 fish oil supplements can reduce impulsivity and hyperactivity.
- Some people report benefits from a complete diet change removing all artificial colourings, additives and unnecessary preservatives.

TIP Improving your child's diet makes sense with a condition such as ADHD, where every boost to health is an advantage. Some parents have found that nutritional therapy can be very informative to get ideas that help you in the right direction with tricky eaters. A dietician will review your child's diet and create a unique diet tailored to his needs. You can find a therapist through the British Association of Nutritional Therapists (www.bant.org.uk; 0870 606 1284).

Sleeping

Sleeping badly is a common problem for children with ADHD, who need at least as much sleep as other children of their age, but tend not to get it, as attention problems can lead to over-stimulation and consequent trouble falling asleep. In turn, lack of sleep can make ADHD problems worse.

Children with ADHD may get up over and over again after you have put them to bed, and have interrupted sleep patterns in the night. Sleep can also be adversely affected by medication, which is a cruel twist when poor sleep is already a problem. There are various strategies that you can try to help with this.

- Have a consistent bedtime, as early as is possible.
- Cut down on television time, especially close to bedtime as television and computer games can have a stimulating effect.
- Increase play and exercise levels during the day to try to tire your ADHD child.
- Cut out the caffeine all day – remember that cola drinks and chocolate have significant amounts.
- A hot, milky drink before bed can be soothing.
- A hot bath before bed can provide relax and chat time – and some parents recommend salts in the bath.
- Have a quiet time for an hour or so before bedtime when colouring, reading, quiet play, stories and cuddles are the main event.

- Try lavender scent in the bedroom, as it can have a calming effect.
- Relaxation tapes such as calming music or nature sounds may make a good background to help your child fall asleep. Some ADHD children find white noise, from an electric fan, or a radio on static, helpful.

> 66 *When Ben was three we went on a family holiday to the mountains. One day we went for a very long walk to a 3,000m peak – which is high for anybody – and back. It took about eight hours, we had a barbecue and we put Ben to bed with the story tapes he always had to go to sleep – and he just wasn't tired. I realised that that was strange, but it was quite typical of the child he was. He never used to sleep in the afternoons or anything like that.* 99
> **Ben's mum**

Sally's story

Sally is 25 now. She was a textbook case of ADHD from birth, but sadly, as her mum Victoria explains, they had not written the textbook then, and it was a long, painful time before they got a diagnosis and help:

Sally was a difficult baby right from the start: she wouldn't feed, she was too angry, too awkward and she was crying too much. She wouldn't sleep a lot and when she woke up she was angry because she was hungry, but because she was angry she was too busy screaming to feed. At night when she woke she was very hard to settle, but when I tried to explain the problem to health visitors they would just patronise and say that we would settle into a routine in time. So I thought it was just us. It was only when I had her little brother and he did sleep and feed and find a routine that I realised how wrong things had been with Sally.

She was quite small when she had to be taken out of her cot because she would escape, and even though we had pillows and mattresses around the landing area there was still a danger that she would hurt herself. So we tried to teach her to sleep on a mattress on the floor without a cot. You couldn't leave her unless she was asleep because it wasn't safe, so I would put her to bed and sit in the room with her without interacting until she went to sleep, which could take two hours. She used to fall a lot and hurt herself; because she wasn't sleeping she was overtired to the point where she was unsteady, and we were often at the hospital where they used to ask us questions about why she was injured so often.

The first diagnosis of any kind was a psychologist who said it was motor impulsivity. You have to imagine that in any situation your brain is always receiving signals, and she finds it impossible to prioritise. So she might be thinking 'What am I going to have for tea tonight?' and there is a ball on the other side of the road, and she cannot think of the consequences of crossing the road – as in there might be a bus coming – because she is thinking about the fish fingers and the ball. By then, at age five or six, she was no different to a two- or three-year-old who you might expect to behave that way.

We were told to be consistent, be firm, and set clear boundaries, which we tried to do though it didn't make much difference. When Sally threw tantrums, which she did in spectacular fashion, she would bang her head on our stone floor and her forehead was permanently bruised. She only stopped when we started laughing at her and saying that it was like going into a bank with a gun and saying 'If you don't give me the money I am going to shoot myself'. That made her realise that it didn't work but she caused herself quite a lot of pain just because of the festering anger and the frustration.

The breakthrough came when my sister read an article in the *Daily Mail* about hyperactivity, which was pretty unknown at that time, and she sent it to me. And I researched it a bit and got on to the ADHD Society which was in its early stages and they sent me some literature. I suppose having failed to get anywhere so many times before I wasn't very optimistic.

A new GP referred us to a child psychologist who specialised in the condition. I was wary of the word psychologist, but we went and saw her and spent half an hour with her, and she confirmed that it was ADHD and recommended Ritalin. Though we were worried about giving Sally mind-altering drugs at the age of six we were desperate to sort out some of her problems.

Ritalin gave Sally the ability to think before she acted; she could sleep and her school work improved. After about a year the

continued

continued from previous page

doctors wanted her to have a break from the drug for one week. Only the school head knew about it. Immediately there was a huge change in her behaviour – she was clumsier and more destructive and disruptive, and the teachers all started asking what was the matter with her. She went straight back on to the Ritalin, and stayed on it till she was 15. There were concerns about her growth – she was weighed and measured a lot. The dose was adjusted up and down. Ritalin really settled her in her later time at primary school. They understood her and she knuckled down quite well with work, and four girls in her year became good friends.

A characteristic was Sally's desperate quest for praise and for acceptance. Once when she was at school we got the dreaded phone call to come and get her. She had been with a group of girls who were quite popular and whose acceptance she really wanted. They had the bright idea that it would be very funny to set fire to the curtains. It had not worked but they had told Sally they would be her friends if she would hide the matches. So with the promise of acceptance, she had done it. The school knew that it just wasn't her style, but as she was caught with the matches the rule was that she had to be suspended. She was victim to so many of those scenarios. It was hard to watch it happening but you couldn't make it better.

At secondary school she boarded, and loved it. She enjoyed being in an environment where there were a wide range of organised activities and sports, it gave her a chance to find things she was good at and shine. She also liked being part of a community where although she lacked a best friend she had enough friends not to be lonely, whereas at home we could never persuade other girls her age to come round. She also benefitted from a structured environment. At home getting her to do homework would have been almost impossible but at school it was in a controlled environment where everyone was working together so there were fewer distractions.

Her medication was dispensed by the matron, and winding matron up became her manipulative game. She still pushed the boundaries but was more manageable. She loved doing well, and it was a huge thing to her if she did. She was sporty and represented the school in all the teams. She was good at maths and science and was always seen as bright, but not taking full advantage, always trying to do things her own way, testing and challenging the rules. She could never take the easy way. She had a group of good friends, but not best friends, and she was never the focus of the group. She became an obsessive emailer and mobile phone user.

Sally still has the tendency towards obsessive behaviour. Also she can be fiercely loyal, which is hard to say when sometimes she has been very disloyal to us. She is very non-judgmental. Now she is older she is good with people and understands their problems. Though she is still rubbish at sorting out her own, she can help other people and likes doing so, and her basically sweet nature has more of a chance to shine through.

6

Dealing with behaviour and other daily difficulties

In the last chapter we looked at practical strategies to help you deal with your child's behaviour. In this chapter, we'll focus on how ADHD could affect him — his social skills and self-confidence.

While it often feels like an uphill struggle, or a fight between you and your child, he will also be confused by his own actions, and upset that he cannot control them. This can directly impact on his self-confidence. His behaviour can also alienate his peers, as other children struggle to be friends with the boy who can't sit still, or parents don't want their child to be friends with the naughtiest boy in the class. We'll look at how you can help improve your child's social skills, and build his confidence.

Making friends and improving social skills

66 *Friendships have started to be an issue for him lately, because of his ADHD behaviour. When he was at nursery he had a massive group of friends because the kids at that age were very hyper anyway, so though he was different the other kids could handle him. Now he is at school with the same kids he has grown up with but where they are calming down he isn't. If he is playing with his friends and he gets over-excited, he can't calm himself down and he ends up lashing out and hitting and hurting them and he doesn't mean to do it. Sometimes he is just a kid fighting with his friends like they all do, but sometimes he just gets so overwhelmed with himself that he lashes out and it is really affecting his friendships. We are hoping that starting on the medication will help before he gets really alienated.* 99
Charlie's mum

Friendships can be a real problem for the ADHD child, as however much he wants to be friends with someone, his behaviour can drive other children away. Reading social cues can be hard for him; he may talk too much, interrupt too much or come over as aggressive or intense. Often he will be emotionally immature compared to other children the same age. This may make him a target for teasing — and he will respond very badly to that. Obviously you want to help your child, and there's a lot you can do in terms of teaching him how to act with other people.

- If you are able to start from a very young age, invite other children round for tea and supervise things more than you would with other children. Get them to play games, and if you notice aspects of your child's behaviour that bother the others talk to them about it afterwards to see if, between you, you can work out ways to modify it.

- Invite only one or two children at a time, preferably at about the same stage with language and physical skills as your child.
- Keep playtimes short, so that your child is less likely to get over-excited and lose control. Try not to plan social activities when he is likely to be tired, for instance after school.
- Be very strict about a no hitting, pushing and shouting policy.
- Praise and reward good social behaviour and emphasise the things he got right.
- If he doesn't quite seem to get how to talk to other children try to teach him a few simple conversation starters, like asking 'What's your favourite game?' and then asking if they want to play it together.
- Try some simple role-playing of social occasions with him.
- Outdoor games and activities such as trampolining can work with other children, but do keep an eye open to check he is playing fair and not getting too over-excited.
- Joining things such as swimming clubs, cubs or brownies, drama or music groups can really help, but stick to the activities he really enjoys. Forcing the pace will almost certainly be counter-productive.

It can be really heartbreaking to see your child struggle with making friends. Another route is to approach other parents, and explain your situation. If he is willing, ask if your child could go round to play, and offer to accompany him so that the strain is not on the other parent to make your child behave.

Building confidence

Life can be full of hard knocks for a child with ADHD, whose behaviour can put him in the frontline for criticism. Many children with ADHD spend a lot of time struggling to fit into a box that is the wrong shape for them — going to school, trying to behave and concentrate and conform. The struggle can easily destroy the child's self-esteem, so it is really important to find things that he enjoys and can do well and encourage them. This is where some of the positives of the condition can come into play — if you can harness some of that energy and enthusiasm into meaningful activity.

> 66 *He has always been the sort of boy who is in all the school plays, bands, scouts, you name it — even when he was young he was at school late every night and it made him really happy. I think that may be a plus side of the hyperactivity — and it continued right through A levels. He is interested in a wide range of things, he loves being active and has far more energy than anyone I know; and he will hurtle around from one activity to another and enjoy them all. That is the very positive side of the condition.* 99
> *Hugh's mum*

Some things — sport, art, dancing, acting — are easy to identify, and it is great if you can encourage your child by enrolling him in teams, groups or extra classes and watching him play or perform. With other children, the talent may be harder to find, but it is worth digging. Perhaps your child is good at collecting things, or sewing, cooking or gardening, mending things or building things, writing stories or poems, entertaining younger children. If there is something, anything, that he is good at and will persevere with and be praised for, it may do wonders for his self-esteem.

> 66 *I love music and drama and creativity. I love writing my own songs and playing them and everything like that but I find it really hard to get my teeth into something. When I play guitar or sing a song my mind is pretty blank. That is like pure silence and that is the most wonderful, happy, relaxed place. I know from being creative with music that I do have that place.* 99
> *Hugh*

Obsessions

Getting completely obsessed with something can be part of the ADHD behaviour pattern, and where other children may stop and start something these children may have a strange, over-focused intensity, which has been described as an attention surplus rather than an attention deficit.

> 66 *Ben once spent an entire day building a K'nex roller coaster from a kit. Other children might have dipped in and out, but his focus was phenomenal, and that is strange in itself. He becomes hyper-focused, gets absolutely obsessed with something and then when it is finished starts jumping around or moves on to the next obsession. At one time he got obsessed with those tiny electric kids' bikes. He was always collecting things from skips, and he managed to do that with bikes, putting them together from scrap, that is the mad, enthusiastic side of him. This hyper-focus is not normal either, it is a weird type of concentration. The other side of that is if he is not interested in something he just can't do it.* 99
> *Ben's mum*

> 66 *Hugh has great perseverance and determination — I don't know if that is a characteristic of ADHD or just him. One example, when he was younger he was obsessed with getting a unicycle. He nagged us and nagged us until we found him one, and then he just kept on doing it until he was good at it because he wanted to.* 99
> *Hugh's mum*

> 66 *If Sally found something she was good at — tennis was an example — she would give it everything. She became one of the school's better players, so everyone wanted to be her partner. She played tennis obsessively because everything was obsessive with her, but it was a positive thing that kept her busy in the summer and got her recognition because she played for the school.* 99
> *Sally's mum*

How to help your child with ADHD

Be aware that obsession is part of the ADHD child's normal behaviour. The best thing, really, is to be flexible enough to allow for eccentricities that do no harm, and can just be part of your child's quirky personality. Go along with and even encourage the positive aspects of an obsession if you can, while trying to keep it within bounds.

Patrick's story

CASE STUDY

Patrick, 11, is not a classic ADHD child in that he could not be said to be developing normally in other ways, and does not have an age equivalent IQ. His mother, Siobhan, is a former nurse:

Patrick has complex needs and a combination of developmental disorders. His autism and his learning difficulties are greater difficulties than his ADHD. However, his level of compulsivity and impulsiveness does make it very difficult for him in the classroom and so it was decided to try Ritalin. We have in the recent past had him on Ritalin but not to huge effect, which is apparently quite common with an autistic diagnosis.

He is now at a school for children with high-functioning autism. He has been there a year and a half and we are still singing its praises. It was only when we got there and we felt confident in the school and the expertise of the staff that we were willing to give Ritalin a go, not least because there is such bad press about it. Initially, certainly, the school would have said Ritalin was a wonder drug for Patrick. So for a child who found it very difficult to sit down and was running out of the classroom a lot and didn't adhere to what was expected of him because he just didn't get it, but also presumably because he had a need to get up and wander around, I think it certainly did calm a lot of that down.

We didn't put him on it to make our lives easier but simply to give him the best possible opportunity to learn at school. Patrick cannot communicate how the Ritalin made him feel, so we were operating completely in the dark. We don't know how things feel for Patrick. He is verbal, but completely unable to express something complex and to do with how things make him feel. The extent of it for him was simply telling him that it was a medicine to help him concentrate, but I don't know what he understood by that.

continued

continued from previous page

Currently he is not on it. The teacher, interestingly, says that without it perhaps Patrick's level of compulsivity and impulsivity is raised a bit. But he has been at the school over a year, long enough to know the score and the behavioural structures and strategies they use, and he understands what he is working towards. The familiarity of the routines at school mean that he is more inclined to go along with it whereas, when he was new, he didn't know what was expected of him. The teacher also said that he felt that Patrick is a bit more open to learning now. He said that he felt Patrick had been zoning out a bit before and now it feels as if you can get through to him a bit better. All I can say is that for Patrick the Ritalin experience has been a bit negligible, and what was too difficult was his not being able to get to sleep until after midnight while he was taking it.

Because he is verbal and quite sociable Patrick is confusing. He comes over quite well and somehow covers up and hides the extent of his learning difficulties — which are severe. What is difficult is that our expectation of him and other people's expectation of him is much greater than he can match up to. He can read and write but at age 11 he still can't do 2+2 and is happy to sit and watch Peppa Pig or sing the Teletubbies theme tune.

As a former specialist nurse, I rate specialism and I find it lacking in a lot of areas to do with special needs children. There seems to be a huge gap between the people who are hypothesising about care and the reality where it hits, and, as a parent, it gets very frustrating. You meet these people when you have just got a diagnosis, which is often at age three or four, and the child development team is all for pre-school under fives, so you meet them and they are gone in a flash. I didn't find them hugely helpful, but it was really too early. You are given what feels like an awful diagnosis and it is so shocking and you tend to react against bad news.

The help offered by social services is a very hard system to get in to and we were allocated inappropriate people and had to tell the same story over and over. These systems are meant to be useful and are not worth having unless they are useful to us. Having one consistent person is very helpful but you do have a problem finding someone who has experience of children right through to adulthood and can give you some idea of what you can expect as your child gets older.

We were referred to a team who are a bit like the child development team but for older children and for children who fall into the severe bracket. Of course you hate the word 'severe' being attached to your child.

Patrick seems very happy at his special school where the staff really seem to know what they are doing. It took a huge change in our thought to go for a special school, but that was part of wanting to deny that that was what he needed, and going there certainly seems to have been the right decision.

7

Impact on the family

66 *ADHD is a family issue, which is why I like to work with both parents. In my experience fathers often tend to be less engaged in the minutiae of day-to-day life, while mothers seem to be the ones who worry more about the impact of ADHD on school work. In a competitive education system they worry that their child may not make the grade. Then mothers have concerns about play dates, where the child doesn't get invited because of their behaviour and they can lose friends. For the child all this can spiral into issues of self-esteem, which is often a factor in ADHD.* 99
Jeremy Monsen, educational psychologist

Siblings

If you have other children, they will undoubtedly feel the impact of having a brother or sister with ADHD. As well as being present during your battles with behaviour, they may also see the amount of time and attention their sibling gets, and resent this. Outings may be limited or end in tears, and levels of family stress may get pretty high from time to time. A child with ADHD's siblings may bear the brunt of his bad behaviour as the child vents his frustration and hyperactivity.

Ideally, siblings need to understand what ADHD is and how it affects their brother or sister as soon as they are of an age to understand it. Explaining about ADHD – in a matter-of-fact way with younger children, with more detailed discussion for older ones – is a chance to talk about their worries and helps them to understand why the sibling with ADHD may be treated differently.

> 66 Sally got desperately jealous, especially of her younger brother. I remember one night when they had both gone to bed and he got up with a sore tummy and I brought him downstairs to sit on my lap. She got wind of this and came hurtling down the stairs at such speed that she put both hands on the wood-burning stove and burned her hands badly because her one focus was that he was there and she wasn't. 99
> Sally's mum

If siblings don't have the condition themselves it can be hard for them to understand why the brother or sister who does can behave so differently and is treated differently. They need to realise that some behaviour relates to the ADHD and is not strictly personal. They can find themselves in situations that they find awkward or embarrassing, such as when the ADHD child has a major tantrum in the supermarket or behaves badly on the bus, and while they often may seem to be coping very well they may also be bottling up their feelings. It can be even worse for them if they are aware that their parents are struggling to cope, as this can make them feel insecure.

> TIP Sometimes family therapy can help you to talk through issues that don't get discussed at home. Therapists can help family members to find better ways to deal with disruptive behaviour and understand each other better.

Birth order

Birth order can affect the impact of ADHD within the family. If the sibling with ADHD is older, the younger ones will never have known any different, and may struggle to understand what is normal behaviour; if younger, your older child or children may resent the disruption, and in turn feel guilty about this resentment.

As the youngest in the family Hugh was always seen as a live-wire with some endearing eccentricities, and it was a long time before it seemed that there was anything of more concern going on.

> 66 He is the youngest of three and I think that may
> be partly why we didn't pick up on the ADHD for a
> long time. It seems quite usual for the youngest to get
> involved in everything, and to be incredibly talkative
> and lively in order to make a bit of an impact within the
> family, and in that way he is a typical youngest child. 99
> **Hugh's mum**

In contrast, Sally, the oldest of three, suffered badly from insecurity, and was jealous of attention given to her two younger brothers even though she was fond of them.

> 66 When her brother was a baby and she was a
> toddler we had to be very careful, because she was so
> impulsive I could never really be sure that she wouldn't
> harm him. She was jealous but it was more [in the]
> little stages when he was trying to pull himself to his
> feet and she would be tearing around with the toys
> flying everywhere. The jealousy was a constant factor,
> but later she was obsessed with what her brother
> was doing at school to the extent that she couldn't
> concentrate on what she was supposed to be doing
> herself. She has always been close to me to the point
> of trying to drive a wedge between me and her father
> and brothers. 99
> **Sally's mum**

Ben's mother, Alex, has seen the damage that one child with ADHD can do to the structure of a family.

> 66 The stress all this creates in a family is so enormous. His sister has phenomenal coping mechanisms. She has been through so much in the last few years, with police coming round and all sorts of things, and him screaming and being violent and breaking things in the house although he is never violent to people. She has had to experience all that but she is amazing. She is a totally different child to her brother, though they are the spitting image of each other, despite the fact that they are not genetically related [see Ben's story, p113]. The problems that ADHD has brought in its wake have impacted on her a lot, though she deals with it all very well. 99
> **Ben's mum**

Patrick's considerable problems mean that his much younger sister does not see him in the pattern of a traditional big brother, and has had to make a lot of adjustments at a young age.

> 66 Patrick's sister is five years younger than him and, strangely, that is OK because up to this point he has been happy to go along with her interests. He does adore her in his way, but he is very unpredictable – he is too rough with her and he can't play with her. He is, I have to say, a constant disappointment to her – she wants more from him. They can't play a game together; if they are out in the garden he will push her over. Over her five years she has learned very cleverly that if she screams, Mummy will come running – and of course I do because I don't trust him either. She is fond of him and is starting to be old enough to understand that there is a reason behind the way he behaves. But at her age things are black and white, good or bad, and as far as she is concerned Patrick is naughty a lot of the time. She witnesses so much of my having to step in and

control him and say no, and things that come to her spontaneously that just don't come to him at all. I suppose she just sees it as him being told off. **"**
Patrick's mum

A lot of children with ADHD are young for their age, and that can invert the natural pecking order in the family. Sometimes, the extra attention that can be focused on the child with ADHD can lead to resentment among siblings.

" Charlie and his little brother Alfie just scrap like normal brothers, though I think Alfie gets jealous of all the attention Charlie has had lately because he has just started on medication. Charlie is very young for his age, and although he is three years older than Alfie his little brother normally bosses him around. Charlie really dotes on his baby sister – all little babies really and he is surprisingly gentle with them. **"**
Charlie's mum

The family situation does have an enormous impact on the child, and it is important to look at the context in which the behaviour occurs and also at the family.

" Children are not treated the same within families. Birth order has an impact, gender has an impact and also whether the parents actually like the child has an impact. Even though they are in the same family, you cannot make the assumption that two children have the same parenting. **"**
Jeremy Monsen, educational psychologist

Two sets of rules?

" I feel like I run with two sets of rules. A set of rules for my daughter, which are quite high expectation in terms of discipline and what is right and wrong, and

then a much lower bar for Patrick, because he can't possibly achieve what I expect for her. I have to get over to her more and more as she gets older that Patrick is different but he is still special and we are all equal, whereas at the moment I think she sees it as me and her against him. Simple things like sitting at the table eating dinner – my expectation is that she sits, eats and stays put and that she finishes what is on her plate, whereas her brother is up, down, up, down and his diet is relatively limited. He refuses most vegetables and that sort of thing. 💬
Patrick's mum

Managing anger

Anger can be a problem for both the ADHD sufferer and his family. Your child with ADHD may be extremely frustrated by the way he feels, and feel out of control. This can be expressed as anger – and vented towards you, or his siblings.

In turn, living with a child with ADHD may cause your other children to feel angry – with them, the situation, and you. There are various techniques that you can teach your children to use to manage their anger (and you might find them useful yourself sometimes).

The first thing is to know what you are dealing with, and the type of anger your child feels is very much a part of their personality. Some children tend to brood, and let their emotions fester away inside, while others will have a violent explosion of rage that will quickly be over. ADHD children are more likely to be in the latter camp anyway, so if you have two explosive types in the house, anything that may help to calm things down will be welcome.

The child without ADHD may get angry with the constraints caused by their sibling's behaviour – not having friends round very much, fewer family outings, feeling that they miss out on attention. It may help if you tell them that it is all right and understandable if some things make them feel angry; it is how they express their anger that can be wrong. Make it clear to them that shouting, hitting and being mean are off limits, especially for everyone who has the advantage of *not* having ADHD. Help them to work out the things that make them angry, talk about how to avoid those things and then suggest some things they could try as ways of dealing with angry feelings when they do happen.

- Go for a fast walk or a run, stamp and jump in the garden, punch a pillow: any sort of physical activity like this is good.
- Put on some loud music (perhaps with headphones for this one unless you want to provoke more anger in other people) for a short time only.
- Talk to someone – mum or dad, a friend, the dog – about being angry, or write it down.
- Have a soothing soak in the bath.
- Stretch out on the floor on their back, and breathe deeply and slowly, or count backwards from 35 to zero; even counting up to 10 under your breath can help.
- Go into a different room, away from the scene of the conflict.

> TIP Making yourself into a kind of anger-management role model for all your children can help you to avoid showing anger to your ADHD child – and some of the techniques may rub off on them.

Your relationship

Understandably, dealing with a child with ADHD can put a strain on your relationship with your partner.

Most two-parent families sometimes quarrel about the best ways to discipline their children, or get annoyed with each other if one of them goes against the rules that they have agreed on, or doesn't follow through with discipline. Adding ADHD into the mix will heighten any of these natural tensions.

To ensure you are a support for each other, communication is key. Don't bottle up how you are feeling – make sure you talk every day, and share what you are struggling with.

- Ensure you are both in agreement when it comes to discipline and rewards. Make your actions consistent.
- Discuss how you are feeling – if you're angry with your partner, explain why; and if you're angry with your child, talk to your partner about it. They may be feeling the same, and this will make you feel less isolated.
- Seek help if you need it. A relationship counsellor may be able to help you talk through some of the problems.
- Remember to have fun together. Family life can be all-encompassing, and extremely tiring. But to have a healthy relationship, it's important to spend time together away from the children. Try to go out for an evening together – even if it is just for a walk – and get family or friends to babysit. Even a short trip out for a coffee can make a difference.

> **TIP** *Special Needs Child: Maintaining Your Relationship* (White Ladder, 2009) focuses solely on this issue. It includes the experiences of other parents who have special needs children, the challenges they have faced and advice on how to overcome them.

66 *Sadly, Ben's relationship with his dad has completely disintegrated. His dad could not cope with his behaviour at all. I think it is the feeling of lack of control over a situation. If your child never does what you say, no matter how much input and support you give, how much counselling you have, how many courses you go on, and you still have problems, in the end it can lead you to despair, and it has been the end of our family as a unit.* 99
Ben's mum

Ben's story

*Ben is 16. His ADHD has caused massive problems throughout
his education, and has made life very difficult for his family as
well. His mother is a teacher who has worked for more than
20 years at a busy, demanding inner-London primary school,
so she knows all about the many and varied challenges which
children can present. Still, her adopted son Ben, now 16, has
tested her almost to the limit:*

We adopted Ben when he was a year old, and his sister, who is
not genetically related to him, when he was four. He was an
adorable baby; very articulate from early on very sociable, an
early talker. He didn't have many tantrums but the ones he had
were enormous. He was very popular at nursery because he was
a lovely kid to have about, bright and quick on the uptake and
he loved all the running around and activity. His very high energy
levels meant that I did try to keep him very busy and made him
incredibly hard work to be around.

When he went to primary school he got into a lot of trouble
in reception and year one because he couldn't sit still on the
carpet at all, he was so restless. But by that age – five – he was
practically reading Harry Potter books. He always just read, from
about the age of three, just picked up a book and read it. So at
that stage I put the trouble down to boredom because he was
ahead of everyone else in the class. But then when he got to
year one there was trouble with his attention. His teachers really
liked him though and they didn't flag anything up and thought
that when he was difficult it was because he was so bright. In year
two he had a bit of a clash with his teacher, and at home I was
increasingly aware that he couldn't do things that were asked of
him, except on his own terms – not wouldn't, couldn't.

He used to play a lot of sport – he was highly gifted at racquet
sports and he used to play a lot of tennis and up until he was

continued

continued from previous page

about nine, the matches were very quick – up to 10 points and that was it. Until then he was at national level and he was winning everything, he was heading for the top and he was really talented. As soon as he had to start playing full sets in tennis that was it. He just couldn't concentrate and his game degenerated to nothing. Because he had been so good it was such a shame. Each time it got to the point in a match where he had to do some thinking he just couldn't do it. Together with his coach we tried everything, all sorts of strategies, nothing worked. Ben started going mad on the tennis court, just going ballistic because he wanted to be winning but he just had no strategy to make it happen.

It was the same with homework – everything would be fine and then we would come to a question he had to think about and he just couldn't do it. I gradually realised that it wasn't that he was being lazy – it was more that he didn't seem to have the thinking processes. When I tried to talk to the school about what was going on with him the reply was that they thought he was just lazy and couldn't be bothered.

Then when Ben was about nine, I read about ADHD. There was a list of symptoms and I realised that he did all of the things on the list, all of the time. Apart from aggression – although he has become verbally aggressive since he hit the teenage years.

I took him to a centre at Horsham to be tested and they confirmed that he definitely had ADHD. They do have to base a lot of the diagnosis on what a parent tells them because when they are testing in a one-to-one situation in a quiet place that is not replicating the conditions of everyday life and the child may well react differently. What was nice was that he used to love going to that centre, even until recently, and he really got on with the doctor.

So I went back to school with his diagnosis and then in year six his behaviour started to deteriorate and he started getting into trouble at school. He wasn't concentrating as they wanted him to for SATS so we decided to try Ritalin, and as soon as he had that he was fine for the whole of year six. However, after that, we did have problems, in that he was fine when he was taking Ritalin, but when he came off it he would have a big wobble and he was having what are called 'downers'. His behaviour could be even worse than before, or he would start crying uncontrollably. They tried varying the prescription around over time, but nothing made it better.

He has never liked Ritalin. He says that it takes away his electricity, and makes him feel as if he doesn't want to talk to anybody. He becomes unsociable, really it takes his personality away. He has recently started saying that he wants to take Ritalin again as he wants to try for some GCSEs and it would be great if it did help now. He may be able to cope with it better now he is older, and actually wants to take it and understands it more. It is a bit less of a worry now he is older because he has done lots of growing already and he is pretty tall. It is good that he wants to get out of the black hole he is in and have a life, and he knows that to do that he needs to have his GCSEs.

He really loved the new independence of secondary school, and he was out late all the time with friends. Then he started to get unhappy with our attempts to keep him within bounds – he was still only 12 – and from that time on he changed. His attitude got worse and worse and for about two and half years he was trying to hang around with the worst crowd in Hackney, and started getting in with the gang culture because he thought that was a really good thing to do. What they saw was a middle-class boy trying to be a gangster and he didn't realise that, because that wasn't how he saw himself. He would do things for them, because it was risky, and he found risk very attractive, and whatever we

continued

continued from previous page

did, however we talked to him, whatever we tried, everything just started to fall to bits from that point.

By this time he had had a few problems in school – including a major tantrum where he had to be held down by teachers and managed to be knocked out. Even after all that, no one at the school ever suggested referring him or trying to get more help. So then I went to the GP and said we needed some help and I got him to refer us to CAMHS. The ADHD was a huge factor, also the fact that he is adopted, which is a massive issue for him.

Because I am a teacher and understand the system and how it works I have been able to go into battle on Ben's behalf. Without me and what I have been able to do for him, I am pretty sure that he would be in prison by now. The worst thing has been him getting into criminal activity which started when he was 13. He has been arrested for a number of things, including burglary. He used to hang around with older boys all the time and they pulled him into trouble. I was always trying to keep him in the house, but you just couldn't ground him he would just jump out of the window and go. He is not at all violent but he was involved with the wrong boys and he was getting involved in really bad stuff, partly because risk is so attractive to some boys with ADHD.

Ben is moving away from his old friendship group but what has happened is that they now don't like him because he has turned his back on them and what they stand for, and as a result he has had a couple of really awful things that have happened. They have a real gang problem at his school and one of the boys came up to him and punched him so hard that it broke his jaw in two places and he had to have a major operation to have that fixed.

One of the unwritten laws is that you don't talk about the gangs, and the kids know it. But Ben said something that was taken as a slight on the gang and which most children just would not say.

It got back to the gang, and that is how he ended up in hospital. He can't help himself, he just says what he thinks and he doesn't have the ability to think 'someone will be angry'. It is such an ADHD thing, speaking without thinking.

After all this, Ben would not go back to school for ages but eventually we persuaded him. He was getting quite a lot of support and I think they actually felt sorry for him for once. They knew he wasn't a fighter; they were very shocked and sad that he had been attacked in the school corridor. He was still finding school very boring and so he used to bunk off a lot, but he was mainly there, working on his GCSEs and really starting to turn a corner. Because he is so clever he would do virtually no work and then they would do a module and he would come really close to getting an A. They were beginning to realise that he is a very bright kid.

Then one night, a group of boys, some of them from the gang at his school, dragged him into an estate and beat him up and made him take his clothes off and do sit-ups and press-ups and said they would put it on Facebook. That was the most horrible and humiliating experience for him, and he refused to go back to school after that.

It has made him very depressed and he talks about all sorts of awful things. He says his life is so terrible and he doesn't know why so many awful things happen to him. He doesn't take responsibility for himself and his actions, and it has taken a long time for him to start understanding that if he does something there will be consequences.

His dad just couldn't handle it. We have separated now and I know that the stress of all this was almost like a bereavement in our relationship. We were both really good, well-behaved children ourselves, and things like having to go to police stations

continued

continued from previous page

and all that is hugely difficult when it is out of your normal life experience. I have had to handle all the problems by myself because I can't walk away. I felt really angry for a long time, now mostly I feel trapped in my life. Home is very difficult. I would like a new relationship but I can't let anyone new into my life because they just wouldn't understand. It is so complicated. It is good in a way that we have moved on, but we are renting at the moment and I am petrified that Ben is going to break up the house if he gets angry. I worry about the neighbours, as they see a boy who flips out and gets angry. Life is very difficult with an ADHD child. No matter how clever he is – and he is – secondary school just hasn't worked out for him.

8

School life and learning

Talk to any parent of a child with ADHD and the one thing that has the potential to cause the most problems is school. If teachers are supportive and helpful, then that is a whole area of worry gone. But this is not the norm, and many parents struggle to get their child the help he needs at school. It's also where children's ADHD can be most obvious and disruptive.

The nature of the condition means that school is the place where children with ADHD have to try hardest *not* to be themselves. This is where you have to sit still, concentrate, behave and fit in – none of which comes easy to a child with ADHD. The policy of including the majority of children in mainstream schools has many benefits, but does mean that any child who does not fit the norm can be seen as a nuisance element. Also, schools often lack the resources and knowledge to do the best they can for these children.

Special schools may be the solution for children with complex needs and more than one condition to contend with, but they are often not suitable for ADHD sufferers.

❝ Hugh was very lucky that he went to the sort of traditional prep school that was very aware that boys need to be active and had them out of doors and dashing around three times a day. He really needed that and he would not have got it at a lot of schools. The other thing that helped him (and I know we were really lucky that this was an option) was that, for his final year at school he became a boarder. This was a massive help organisationally. He had always been the kind of boy who had trouble keeping all his stuff in the right place, and suddenly he had a structured environment and a completely structured day. He still says that he can't work in his room at home as there are too many distractions, and he has to go to a library to work. The other thing about it that was wonderful for him was that he could fill up every hour of the day if he wanted to – and he is a boy who likes to be very busy. ❞
Hugh's mum

❝ I trawled the country to find a special school that would cater for Ben, but what happens is that they are all for very severely disabled or behaviourally disturbed children and so on. There is nothing for children that are not extreme cases but for whom every day is really hard. You need a school that knows that for these children all day, every day in school is going to be a struggle but they are going to go all out to make it successful for them. They just don't seem to exist. Especially not for children who are academically able. There is just no place to go for kids that can't fit into the mainstream system. ❞
Ben's mum

The reality is that teachers are not trained to manage specific problems, such as ADHD. Often teachers have little understanding of ADHD children, and cannot see beyond the problems they create. Class sizes are often 30-plus, with several disruptive children and teachers have no specialist training in how to deal with them.

Such situations are fair to no one. Statistically there will be at least one child with ADHD in the class, and with no understanding and support, his behaviour will be disruptive for everyone.

Greater understanding, and more attention to helpful strategies, would almost certainly improve the classroom situation for everyone.

> 66 *School teachers have not tended to have much general training in these areas of child development, and even if this is changing now it probably does not affect older teachers who would not have had much on ADHD and autistic spectrum disorders if they trained even a decade ago. With the tendency towards inclusivity I feel that part of the teaching curriculum should include general training in child development, what is normal and what is not. The more modern-thinking services are starting to do more training in schools, so that teachers might pick up that there is something amiss with the child – and then they would refer the child to the educational psychologist, who might then make an assessment.* 99
> *Dr Dinah Jayson*

Finding a smallish school, extra teaching support, a special needs teacher for some aspects of learning or a specialist ADHD tutor for after school seems to work well for the lucky ones who are able to access this through the mainstream system. But getting this help can be an uphill struggle. See p126 for the official steps you can go through to get support for your child, but first we'll look at what you and his teacher can do to help.

Suggestions for your child's teacher

There are lots of specific techniques and strategies to support ADHD children in their education, and this is an area that is developing all the time. It is well worth talking to your child's teachers to check that they know at least as much as you do. Each student needs different help, and you can help the teachers to work out what specific things are hard for your child.

Every school has a special educational needs co-ordinator (SENCO), who is there to give additional support to children with special educational needs (SEN). Many classes also have a teaching assistant (TA) who is there to give one-on-one attention to the children. Ensure you meet with your child's teacher, the SENCO and the TA to find out what they know about ADHD and if they have any experience of teaching children with ADHD. The TA may be instrumental in your child's learning, and may know the most about what he is like in class and what might help him.

Some students with ADHD may have trouble getting started on a task, others may have trouble finishing one task and starting on the next. Many of them will suffer from the effects of being inattentive – such as forgetting their homework. If you can make sure the teachers know what their problems are it will be easier for them to work out how to help them. It will make a big difference if you establish a good relationship with your child's teacher and encourage them to give you plenty of feedback.

It's important to acknowledge that if your child is extremely hyperactive and disturbs other classmates on a regular basis, his teacher may see him as the 'problem child' in the class. Whatever you can do to help them understand your child more will help everyone involved.

- The teacher needs to be aware that pupils with ADHD are likely to be talkative, demanding and very noticeable in the class. This is how they are, and showing irritation will not make them change.
- Perhaps a younger child who has trouble sitting still could be the 'teacher's helper', tidying up the room, handing things out and so on.

- Clear rules and routines help children with ADHD. It helps if teachers have set times for specific tasks, and draw attention to any changes that are made, making sure that they have registered with the ADHD children.
- Children with ADHD often perform well at short, sharp tasks but have real problems with longer-term projects where they do not have direct supervision, and it can be helpful if the teacher bears this in mind and gives them a bit of extra help if possible.
- Children with ADHD have particular problems with learning by rote, so it will make a difference if the teacher can emphasise study skills and strategies to help them learn crucial basics such as times tables, which some of them find very hard to do.
- The teacher should try to give instructions step by step to make sure that anyone with ADHD can follow them. The directions should be given both in writing and verbally. Students with ADHD may benefit from doing each step as a separate task.
- Teachers can try to help an ADHD child channel their energy with physical activity where they can. They can try giving the child regular breaks, and perhaps let him do some of his work standing up.
- Ask the teacher to provide feedback to your child in private rather than in front of the whole class.
- Boys in particular seem to respond better to praise given one to one rather than in front of others.

> 66 *Charlie has always been as bright as a button and his memory is fantastic. When he started nursery and school he just couldn't manage to sit in one position. Over the last year at junior school, two teachers he has had have been really good. While his behaviour has been erratic they have been able to cope with him because they know what he is like and maybe make a few allowances for his behaviour. On the whole he responds well to praise and they have taken a fairly positive attitude. He is not very keen on his teacher now and I think she is finding it quite hard to handle him, so we have had to have a lot of input with the school.* 99
> **Charlie's grandmother**

One-to-one teaching has been shown to be massively helpful for children with the concentration problems of ADHD, and you may be able to access some of this through School Action (see p127), before having to get a statement.

Schemes such as Volunteer Reading Help (www.vrh.org.uk) operate in some schools. Having someone to help with his reading on a one-to-one basis can transform school life for an ADHD child whose concentration issues may have affected his ability to read and keep up with the class, thereby denting fragile self-esteem.

> 66 *The one-to-one teaching satisfies Emil's need for attention quite apart from anything he learns. I do think there will always be personality issues for him, however much he progresses with his reading. I have only recently discovered that he has ADHD, which his mother is reluctant to address because of the stigma she sees, and this does seem to make sense of the way that he rushes to conclusions and always wants everything to happen right now.* 99
> **Jane M, a volunteer in the scheme**

Undoubtedly, communication with your school is key, and the help and support from a school can make all the difference – both when it comes to recognising ADHD and after it is diagnosed. An understanding head teacher can smooth the path for you and your child.

> 66 *His headmistress is very supportive of him. It came to the point where his mum was always up at the school because of some bit of naughtiness of Charlie's. He couldn't sit down and concentrate, and Lisa, and the school, thought they needed to get to the bottom of it. He is really good at maths and he has a vivid imagination, but since he was little you have always had to keep him really occupied and grab his attention.* 99
> **Joan, Charlie's grandmother**

> TIP Children can struggle to manage their medication regime in the school setting, as the pastoral care they need for this is often not readily available. It is vital that your child's teacher or TA is made aware of what medication your child is on, and when he needs to take it.

How you can help your child in school

There is a lot you can do yourself to help your child in school, and the earlier you start the more difference it will make. It will really help if you make a point of getting to know the teacher and TA at school or nursery, and try to discuss your child and what he needs, to see if you can work together.

- Check where your child sits in the classroom and ask if he can be moved if you think he should be nearer to the teacher, or away from possible distractions.
- Ask for tasks to be broken down to a level that your child can understand, and if the teacher doesn't have time, see if you can do it at home.
- That means keeping an eye on what he is doing in school. If possible, see if you can get a programme of the work he will be doing, so that you know what will be expected of your child and can help him with any clear obstacles.
- Tell him always to ask for help when he doesn't understand something, and, at appropriate ages and stages teach him basic study skills such as reading out loud, note taking, underlining and highlighting work.
- When you are helping with homework keep the subject alive and busy. Talk a chapter of a book through with him. ADHD children often have masses to say if you can keep them interested in the subject.
- Your ADHD child is more than likely to have self-esteem issues, so give him a boost by praising his work and behaviour

whenever you realistically can, and ask the teachers if they can do the same.

- Give him a ball of putty to fiddle with in class (this is acknowledging his need to fidget – part of accepting how he is and adapting).

As a parent you can help with some simple one-to-one strategies out of school, just by talking through what your child did at school every day, and most importantly by being there when he has homework to do. By staying with him you can sometimes do what he cannot do for himself – bring his attention back to what he is meant to be doing, and keep his mind from wandering. If he is left alone to do his homework it can take him forever – and may actually never get finished.

> ❝ I never made a conscious decision to not do the work, but when I was in my room and meant to be getting on with homework suddenly I would become aware that 20 minutes had gone by. I wasn't leaning over the paper with the pen poised to write the first sentence, I was reclining in the chair twiddling the pen between my fingers and with no recollection of how I got to that stage. ❞
> *Hugh*

Accessing help at school

As well as the issues we have addressed already, there are more formal ways to get your child the help and support he needs. The help available varies throughout different local authorities, but could come in the form of a learning support assistant, assigned solely to your child, a specialist teacher who has a brief for emotional and behavioural difficulties that would cover ADHD or specialist ADHD nurses, who conduct home visits and support families. But to access all of this help, you'll have to make your way through the SEN system – a thing that many parents before you have struggled with.

So, how do you access the help that your child needs? How can you make the system work for you, and whose numbers do you need on speed dial in case of difficulties?

The first step along the road to getting your child help at school is to meet with your child's teacher and his SENCO. Every school has a special educational needs policy and code of practice. Ask to see this, as it will show you what procedures they will go through to help your child, and what help they are able to provide.

School Action

After talking with your child's teacher and SENCO, they may decide to put him on the School Action Plan. This is the first step to getting the help you need for your child. The school will create an individual education plan (IEP) for your child, using the internal support systems they have at the school – which might be more attention from the SENCO. IEPs are reviewed twice a year.

School Action Plus

If your child seems to need more help than the School Action Plan gives him, they may be moved up to School Action Plus. If your child's needs are numerous from the outset, they may move straight onto this plan. School Action Plus will involve other health professionals, for example, an educational psychologist.

You may well find it helpful to cultivate a relationship with the educational psychologist, who can be a source of objective advice on strategies to help your child in school. They have massive experience of problem areas, and good working relationships with schools, so they can guide you through difficult and potentially confrontational areas if you feel the school is not doing the best for your child. Sometimes it helps both sides if parents and teachers get together under the guidance of a professional to set clear targets for the child.

66 *Teachers are under a lot of pressure and usually by the time a psychologist is involved they are fairly desperate, they have tried everything and they feel quite stuck. In general I think teachers are torn between the demands of the curriculum, the other children in the class and the stress and pressure that the ADHD causes. I think the will is there and often they are very appreciative of someone coming in and reframing situations, and pointing out the positives in the situation and the things that can be built on.* 99
Jeremy Monsen

Statements

A Statement of Educational Needs (known as a statement) is a legal document which is issued by your local authority – and it can be hard to come by. The statement sets out your child's needs and the help he should have. To obtain a statement, your child needs to undergo an assessment, which can take around six months. This assessment aims to establish what your child's SEN are and comprises reports from the parent, the child's teacher, an educational psychologist, a paediatrician or doctor, and any others who are already helping your child.

> TIP Your child does not have to have been on the School Action Plan to be assessed for a statement. If his needs are severe enough, the school may recommend seeking a statement as the first step.

Once the assessment has been carried out, the information may be fed into a statement. If the assessment finds that your child does not need a statement, they will issue you with a letter, which will detail what other help your child will be provided (similar to the help given on a School Action Plan). You can appeal against this decision through the Special Educational Needs and Disability Tribunal (www.sendist.gov.uk).

The reality of the situation is that whether your local authority will issue a statement to your child doesn't just depend on his needs – it also depends on the local authority's budget. Additional support is expensive, and this sometimes plays a part in the level of help they are willing to provide. It can sometimes be hard to drive a statement through, and if you are struggling with this, enlist the support of the school and all the other professionals who may be involved.

> **TIP** Take notes at every stage of the statementing process, so that if you need to appeal you have all the documentation you need.

The statement is reviewed annually to ensure that any extra support given continues to meet your child's needs.

Tips for parents

- Get a copy of the SEN Code of Practice from the Department for Education and Skills (DfES) (www.dfes.gov.uk).
- Ask to see local authority guidance/policy for SEN.
- Keep copies of all letters and take notes in meetings.
- Keep a diary of your child's progress and the difficulties you encounter.
- Ask for help from Parent Partnership through your local education authority.
- Ring the education board and ask who is dealing with your case.
- Find out your rights in the school and ask to see the SEN policies of the school.
- Read the policies thoroughly and take notes if you need to.
- Don't be afraid to speak out and fight for your child.
- Always ask if you don't know something or don't understand.

The head teacher of an inner city primary school talks about ADHD

You have to go down every route with a child who seems to be showing problem behaviour or having difficulties in school: talk to the parents, talk to the teacher, who would have identified various things that were happening, see if you can mend those things. It would probably be affecting the child's work, so then we call the educational psychologist in and she does all the tests such as IQ tests, visual awareness tests, all these things. She would probably say if she thought it was anything to do with ADHD or autism and would suggest that the child should go to their GP or have a paediatric assessment and that would be the course of action. The initial thing would be working out what affects the child in school. We would take it very seriously, whatever it is, which we do with every child.

It is interesting that at the school we have never received guidelines on how to deal with ADHD. The children I have known where they have said they have ADHD have all been quite different, even if they may exhibit the same things. This school has found a lot of problems, in that, historically, a lot of children who have been diagnosed with ADHD have had parents who have had real problems as well, or there has been something major that has triggered some of the behaviours off. I think it is very complicated. Parents seem to think that it is just because they can't keep still and that it is all very simple, but it is not.

One little boy recently whose mother thought he had ADHD is one that I have watched quite a lot. He was all over the place, up and down all the time and clearly bored in class and now we have put him up a year and we don't hear a peep out of him. He can actually sit very quietly when he is interested in something, and he can sit and do maths very easily with a lot of concentration. Now he is sitting most of the day. It probably wasn't ADHD at all, he just needed to be challenged more with work. I think this type of confusion does happen a lot, and parents will just reach for a label to explain why their child is not fitting in. We watch each child and work things out for them on an individual basis. A lot of where people are getting their information from is television programmes like Super Nanny, where extreme cases make a better show – and usually get sorted out within the hour's programme. I don't think it gives parents a very realistic template.

Another child we had had been at a very formal Catholic school, and it was thought that the way we do things here, which is very tailored to the individual child, might help him. It didn't really work out for him, although we noticed a big difference in him when he started on Ritalin, but then it all fell apart again. I went to visit the referral school where he went and he couldn't fit in even with the individual attention. He has found something to do with football now which seems to be suiting him. His mother used to do everything she could to wear him out – she used to have him manically doing things every night. He used to go swimming most nights, do rugby, something every night, but she could never really get him tired.

We are a school with a very close staff. There are about 28 teachers, most of whom have been here for 20 or more years. It is tough but it is supportive and rewarding. We talk to children a lot. It is quite a happy place but when you have a child that goes over the top it is hard for everyone. Because a lot of the other children are so brittle, if one gets into a state it can ripple through all of them. There are procedures that you have to follow, in some circumstances. I have only ever permanently excluded three children, which is very low for an inner-city area like this. I don't like doing that but the system isn't always very sympathetic to children who are different and who have problems.

Parents often resist the idea of a label such as ADHD, perceiving it as a stigma – for instance, we had a boy who climbed up to the top of an indoor water pipe about 10 feet up and wouldn't come down until his mother came. He clearly had something amiss, but she refused to go down that route and remained convinced that we just weren't working him hard enough in school. But you do get to know when children just aren't conforming to the norm. Sometimes we will offer to go to a psychologist with the child and parent and they will refuse point blank. It is part of a thing where parents would rather have the stigma of their child's bad behaviour than the perceived stigma of a condition, even though you can explain to them that it is not about madness and no blame attaches to them – it makes no difference. If only educational psychologists had a different name with fewer connotations it might help. What is difficult is that these children look bright and healthy generally, there is nothing you can see with ADHD, and you have to find a way to make it clear that it is their behaviour that you don't like, not them.

What to do when there are problems with school

In an educational system which prescribes inclusion in the mainstream for children with a raft of special needs, including ADHD, the lack of provision for these children, and the frequent deficiency in education or support for the teachers who should be dealing with these educational needs as part of their job, can be scandalous. If teachers do not understand, or are not aware of your child's ADHD, they can put it down to extremely naughty behaviour – and blame the parents. The persistent refusal of some teachers and some schools to take the condition seriously can make life even more difficult for families who are already feeling embattled.

❝ When Ben started secondary school I went through all the procedures so that they were informed about his special needs, and we were going along OK. But then in the second term he seemed to be getting more and more unhappy and his behaviour was changing at home. His form tutor said that Ben's behaviour at school was OK, but that he seemed to have difficulties with concentration. When I asked if she knew he had ADHD and was on Ritalin she told me she had no idea. Not one person in that school, apart from the

special educational needs co-ordinator, knew that not only did he have ADHD but that he was on a daily dose of a very high prescription drug to treat it. I was very annoyed by that. The co-ordinator said she had emailed everyone and it was up to them if they read it, and really we had trouble with the school from that point on. That did shock me. 99
Ben's mum

Some parents are put in the horrible situation where the school attempts to get their child suspended or excluded, due to bad behaviour.

66 *One really good thing that CAMHS did was to call someone in to fight our battle at school. He was the region's behaviour specialist. The school was a faith school and not very tolerant, but he was able to come into these endless round table reviews they have in school when they are trying to get rid of your child. He was able to tell them that what they were doing was very wrong, that Billy has this condition and can't help himself, and that they needed to change to accommodate him because he couldn't change to accommodate them. That was really useful. When you talk to parents as I do, they all throw their hands up in horror when you talk about schools. In fairness to them the teachers don't get any training in how to manage kids with ADHD.* 99
Billy's mum, who runs an ADHD support group for parents

If you are coming up against animosity in your school, the best thing you can do is seek external advice. Go to your GP, get in touch with CAMHS or contact the Special Educational Needs and Disability Tribunal (www.sendist.gov.uk). Ben's mum had to take his case to a tribunal, when the school tried to exclude him (see below).

> **TIP** The most helpful thing you can do is to get your child's teacher onside. ADHD behaviour can often be interpreted as naughty and defiant behaviour, and if it is viewed that way by the teacher they are going to be negative in their responses, rather than looking for ways around the problem.

School trips

It pays to be aware that school trips can be a danger area for children with ADHD, away from normal supervision and routine, and parents are wise to approach them with caution. You need to check that all the staff involved know of your child's condition and are confident that they can cope.

Make a list of anything that you think the teachers might need to know about your child and the issues that might arise on the trip; make sure that the teachers (who may not be the ones who know about your child) are aware of medication details, and prepare your child as thoroughly as you can for the experience. Ben's mother did all this, but still experienced a lot of unnecessary worry and expense, not to mention an unexpected trip abroad to fetch him, when he went on a school trip to Italy when he was 12.

> 66 The group had been to an amusement arcade, just the sort of place to get Ben totally over-excited. He won the top prize, which was a penknife and put it in his pocket. One of the other kids told the teacher that Ben had a knife in his pocket and he got into all sorts of trouble. He was done for possession of the knife, and we were summoned to Italy to take him home. The teachers felt he should have known it was wrong to pick a knife as a prize. I felt that, as they had taken the kids to somewhere where the prize on offer was a knife, they might expect someone like Ben to pick it. Other children did worse things, but they were better at hiding them than Ben. 99

66 *They wanted to permanently exclude him from the school. I took it to a special needs tribunal. I got together a massive folder detailing all the things they hadn't done, including the failure to support him in school, all the things that they had got wrong over the trip. It went to the education authority, who advised the school that they were going to lose because they hadn't done what they were supposed to do. So they took him back. Permanent exclusion on such flimsy grounds was draconian. The teachers were questioned as to why they took the children to an amusement arcade. The other boy who had a diagnosis of ADHD who went on the trip also came back permanently excluded, and he was never allowed back. It does not say much for the school's ability to handle such children.* 99
Ben's mum

Billy's story

CASE STUDY

Because he spent time in care before he was adopted and no one really looked at his problems, Billy did not get a diagnosis and medication for his ADHD until he was 15, by which time his educational difficulties were quite severe, as his mother explains:

I think in the care system it is even harder to get diagnosed. Our kids were seven and eight when we adopted them and Billy's ADHD had never been diagnosed although there were clearly signs that no one had picked up. Then we spent five years trying to eliminate other conditions before we could get anywhere with a diagnosis. It is a difficult condition to diagnose and there is sometimes some reluctance. There are other conditions with closely related symptoms. With my son it could have been attachment disorder, and at one time they thought he might be

continued

continued from previous page

autistic. I went through all this for years on end and they saw him endlessly at CAMHS for assessments. Then they eventually decided on ADHD and then he got medication.

My son was extraordinarily challenging – my feeling is that he has oppositional defiant disorder as well. He is not hyperactive but extraordinarily impulsive. He was prescribed slow-release Concerta, and at first he had one during the day at school and then another when he got home which was to help him with his revision. It would have made such a difference if he could have had those tablets from the beginning of secondary school. We didn't adopt him until he was nine, and it was only when he was 10 or 11 that we could have got anything anyway. But if we had been able to start earlier, who knows how much more he could have made of his schooldays? He was always a very bright kid and very outgoing. I can spot them a mile off now. If he had had that medication he would have been able to focus from the first year of senior school. He wouldn't have got into bother, he wouldn't have been chucked out of class all the time and then ended up being sucked into the bad crowd at school.

He is 17 now and it is very difficult. He was very compliant in his last year at school, to the extent that he would come to me and ask for his tablet. Then at 16 in our area you are not referred to CAMHS any more, you get referred to an adolescent unit and now he is at an age where he wants to assert himself, which is double trouble. He feels that the tablets make him unable to eat, which is probably true, and he doesn't like that and he doesn't like the feeling it gives him. So he had a period of refusing to take his tablets, which was a shame because his unregulated impulsive behaviour meant that he got chucked off the apprenticeship he had started. Then he roamed from placement to placement trying to get something. He is now back on half-strength 18mg Concerta, which is next to nothing, and he has just been sacked from another job. I am trying to get him to think about upping the dose again.

I went back to CAMHS because I have helped them to set up
a participation group to help the kids have their say about how
the service should be delivered. A new set of lads turned up for
this group, and it took us about three minutes flat to work out
that these were the kids with ADHD – because their job was to
review a service leaflet and say how it could be bettered, and
they gave it all of about seven minutes and then they completely
lost interest. When I asked if they would read something like that
if it came to their house, they all said no because there were too
many words in it.

I haven't really found anything else that works for Billy apart from
medication, except one thing I learned on the Barnardo's course,
which was the importance of establishing a firm routine, though
in everyday life it is hard to enforce. Billy is in a good family, the
others are all good children, but it is nothing to do with home.
We tried so hard to get him into good activities – things like
scouts, but they had a round of applause when he left there;
he couldn't cope with the marching and the orders at cadets,
couldn't get his head round the sequences.

We did really, really try to get him into things that would help
him. He is very sociable, but like a lot of kids with ADHD, they
don't keep their friends, because they are so high maintenance.
Just lately his dad managed to get him into a football team for
the first time and he likes that. He has met a few people through
that and he is managing to stick to them by not seeing them too
much. We have tried to get him to see each person once a week
as a way of managing his full-on-ness with people. He knows
he is doing it but he can't control it and he wouldn't be able to
articulate it. But I know that he knows deep down that we are
trying to help, but he wants to control things.

They say with people with ADHD that they have to make the
same mistake 19 times to learn from it. I often say to him right
continued

continued from previous page

son you've done this 18 times now is the time to stop. It is said for a laugh, but it really is true. Because he is so impulsive – he has been working in a garage but he wants to wear his best clothes to work. The more we tell him to wear his old things to work the more he insists and he has ruined outfit after outfit.

The other thing that happens particularly in the North, I don't know about the more affluent regions, is the problem with managing money. Billy does get DLA [disabled living allowance] and it goes directly to him though it will be stopping shortly. I control it, and I keep half of it back and that pays for things like all these clothes he keeps wrecking, and half of it goes to him and then he goes out and spends it that night. Even though he knows he will want to buy things like cigarettes during the week he cannot control it at all. As soon as he has got it out it goes, and that is a very typical problem, which I suspect would apply, however affluent the family.

An interesting thing I have discovered through experience is the strong hereditary factor in ADHD, which means that a lot of the parents have it, and it doesn't make trying to organise a parents' support group any easier. At CAMHS the other week they told us he would grow out of it and even Billy looked astonished. It would be wonderful if they were right, but I remain very far from convinced.

9

Growing up
with ADHD
What the future holds

The teenage years can be pretty tough for any parent, but when you add ADHD into the mix you are probably going to experience extra problems. Behaviour issues may have calmed down a lot, especially if you caught them early, but immaturity, attraction to risk and organisational difficulties that go with the territory are hardly likely to make life easier for you or your child.

66 *If I was giving advice to a parent with an ADHD teenager I would say, be prepared for the fact that it will be hard and always bear in mind that your child will probably have difficulties in perceiving consequences. Cause and effect is lost on them. The only thing that has worked on my son is his fear of being in a police cell. He cannot bear to be confined. His behaviour had to get to that low level before he found a deterrent. If you look at the prison population, the proportion of young offenders is hugely people who have issues of this kind, and all the theory is failing them.* 99
Ben's mum

Further education

ADHD is not in itself a definer or limiter of intelligence. Depending on the extent to which educational issues have been brought under control, there is no reason why your child won't be off to university or college with the rest. However, it is only realistic to be aware that problem years in school don't always translate to success in exams, and you will know if you need to be considering other options.

Sadly, a recent study found that teenagers with ADHD are less likely to complete school on time than teenagers with other, often more severe, mental health disorders, with almost one-third of teenagers diagnosed with the combined form of ADHD dropping out or delaying the completion of school.

There is perhaps some comfort to be gained from the fact that a significant number seem to return to their studies in their twenties – possibly because they have become more mature, or have belatedly understood the point of having some qualifications. Your support and understanding are crucial in helping your teenager to stay on track with his studies, and making sure he gets the treatment most suitable for him.

> ❝ Being a teenager is very tough anyway, and if you have all these other things piling in then it really is very hard. We probably spent about £3,000 on the educational psychologist, the psychiatrist and the counsellor. But when you think what it costs when people do go wrong and don't get help then that was money well spent. I just think there must be a lot of other kids who suffer from not getting help. The teenage years are when they are struggling and often when things can turn around and start going right – but equally when they can all start going badly wrong. If you get the right help, as Hugh did, it can turn you around. ❞
> *Hugh's mum*

How ADHD may change

Many children with ADHD continue to have symptoms in adolescence, and some parents discover that their child has the condition for the first time during the teenage years. This is more common among those with mainly the inattentive form of ADHD, because they are not normally noticeable or disruptive at home or school, but as academic demands and responsibilities increase their condition becomes more apparent.

> ❝ Sally is able to accept that she has had a lot
> go wrong in her life. She does not criticise or get
> prejudiced against people and will often see the good
> in them, and I think that is one of her more positive
> things. Although she flits from one thing to another,
> whatever she is doing at the time she will give 110%.
> The trouble is the inconsistency that means that she
> has had so many career choices and always changes
> her mind. When she was younger, she would take up
> all the different sports and activities and get all the kit,
> have the lessons, and then as soon as it went wrong
> it was over. It is low self-esteem and you can't blame
> her for that. I haven't found anything that really makes
> things better for her. ❞
> **Sally's mum**

Hyperactivity tends to decrease as a child gets older, but in teenagers who continue to be hyperactive it may transmit to restlessness and attempts to do too much at once. Teenagers responsible for their own medication may find it hard to stick with treatment. They may have trouble controlling their impulsivity, and may be on a short fuse, so you will find that rules and structure at home are as important as ever. Keeping up with things such as therapy or counselling can help you all during these years.

> ❝ One of Ben's problems was that he had huge
> identity issues because of his adoption. The emotional
> impact of that was huge. Then there is the fact that

*he is very bright – which can be a problem in itself.
Combined with the ADHD and teenage hormones, it is
a really bad cocktail.* 🍸
Ben's mum

You may find that what your child needs in the way of treatment may change as he hits the teenage years, so make sure that you keep up with his medical appointments and press for a review from time to time. If behavioural problems crop up you want to be sure that this is not because the medication needs adjustment.

In general, symptoms may start to diminish as a child grows up, although up to half of children with ADHD will go on having symptoms such as poor organisational skills well into adulthood. All the tools that you can give them to deal with this will help them to make a transition to a more independent life. Keeping discipline, order and consistency at home is paramount. If homework is an issue, you can help by having some kind of a homework contract – but you need to let your teenager have a say in the terms you set out so that it doesn't become a constant battleground. Make sure that the routine focuses on what will work best for them in terms of what topic is done on which night, the timing and where the homework is done. With all this enshrined in routine, it may be easier for your teenager to see that getting the work done at home has benefits, not least in terms of not getting into trouble at school.

Teenagers with ADHD generally mature more slowly than others of the same age, and they will need help to learn the skills for independent living.

- **Time management** is a problem for people with ADHD, who tend to have a badly developed sense of time, of how long things take, and of how much time has elapsed. Encourage your teenager to wear a watch and encourage and reward good time-keeping.
- **Planning and prioritising the day**, establishing which things have to be done at a particular time, working out that some jobs have to be finished before a leisure activity can be enjoyed

is exactly the type of thing that may not come naturally to someone with ADHD. But you can encourage them to have control over their day-to-day schedule while they still have the safety net of home and school accounting for most of their day.

- **Daily routines** are an important aspect of time management. Encourage a teenager with ADHD to work out a routine for morning and evening. This will make things much easier for them and for you.
- **A good night's sleep** is crucial, as sleep problems are very common for ADHD teenagers, and lack of sleep can only increase ADHD symptoms. Encourage your teenager to develop a regular bedtime and try not to get into the habit of being a night-owl.
- It is important to give your teenager the responsibility for waking themselves in the morning, but if that is not going to work, try to be strategic so that the day doesn't start with a battle.

66 *I invented a good ruse for getting the medication sorted out. It involved taking Billy's breakfast up to his room on a tray, at 7am, putting on the television in his room, giving him a cup of tea and his tablet, because it takes an hour to get into the system, and then going away for an hour. I found out the hard way that if I left it till 8am to say 'Here's your tablet, now get up and off to school', then it just wasn't going to happen. By waking him an hour early and giving him the medication while he was still groggy, then leaving him with the television and the breakfast, an hour later I went back to a transformed boy. He would jump out of bed good as gold and wash his face without having to be coaxed through every step.*

It was blissful and I used to think every day what a transformation the tablets had made to our lives because the mornings used to be such a battle to get him up and washed. Everything used to have to be broken down into little steps every single day because

these boys can't hold sequences of instructions in their heads. Billy is not hyperactive but he is particularly affected by that side of it, so it really does have to be one thing at a time. 99
Billy's mum

- **Good food** is essential, but the classic teenage diet of fast food and snacks is full of things that will not do much for someone with ADHD. Serve healthy, nutritious food at home, encourage him to make healthy choices for himself, giving lots of guidance on what these healthy choices should be – and at the same time, don't fret about some burgers and pizzas along the way.
- **Regular exercise** is very important in reducing the impact of ADHD. While organised sport is generally a regular part of schooldays, it does not necessarily feature at college or the outside world. It is worth encouraging your teenager into some form of regular exercise outside school, so that the habit may continue.

66 *In my frustration about feeling I wasn't being given enough information, especially about the future, I kept thinking that there must be some professionals out there who know how things are for a 15-year-old, a 20-year-old and beyond to give me some sort of perspective about what is ahead. I have not really found them yet.* 99
Patrick's mum

Teenage issues

Driving

A lot of teenagers take risks, but those with ADHD, especially untreated ADHD, are more likely to do so. US statistics show that in their first few years of driving, ADHD teenagers are involved in nearly four times as many car accidents as others and get three times as many speeding tickets, and things are unlikely to be very different here. You know your child, and if you think his level of ADHD makes him potentially dangerous behind the wheel then defer the driving lessons until you think he is truly ready. If that day does not dawn, help him to think positively about other ways of getting around.

> 66 Cycling is my choice. I pretty much may put myself in danger but it is only me. The pressure with driving is the instant you get into a car, you are putting lots of other people at risk and I don't trust myself not to get distracted. I think that is enough reason not to become a driver apart from the environmental ones. 99
> Hugh

If your teenager is having driving lessons, make sure that he understands the rules of the road and conforms to them. It is very important that ADHD teenagers have a lot of driving practice under adult supervision, much more than their peers will probably need. When they do pass the driving test you will feel a lot happier if they go on to take the Pass Plus test, which gives them some motorway experience.

Drugs

Unfortunately, the stage where teenagers lose the safety net of school can be very difficult for your ADHD teenager, and you may have to work very hard to keep them on track. There are lots of pitfalls that just seem to fit in all too well with the condition, such as the temptation to 'self-medicate' with recreational drugs and the attraction of anything a bit risky.

> 66 The attraction of the buzz from risky behaviour is a very ADHD thing. Ben has been done for possession of cannabis because he is into smoking it and whatever you tell him about that he doesn't stop. So now he has got quite a serious criminal record and there are a lot of issues about why he is not in school. To be fair to

*him he has tried and tried not to get involved in that
bad kind of activity and to keep away from the gang
culture. He is still doing things he shouldn't do, but is
not harming other people.* 🔊
Ben's mum

For parents vigilance is the key, and it is important to do
everything you can to keep your teenager profitably occupied,
with courses, apprenticeships or further study, really anything
you can find to keep him from sinking into a slough of
unemployment and misery. Support at this stage can be patchy
– once he is 16 he is no longer referred to CAMHS, he may want
to organise things for himself, but this is probably not exactly his
strongest area.

66 *It is so hard for them to find jobs. I won't let Billy just
sit around but it will come to the point where I can't
influence him any longer. Once he is 18 he will get his
£50 or whatever a week dole. At the moment he is very
motivated by money and reward, but if he is getting
£50 a week to not do anything then he will take the £50
a week and not do anything.*

*Everything is stacked against these kids really and I
know from talking to parents of slightly older ADHD
teenagers that this is a common problem. They have
lost confidence from trying and failing to find work over
and over and they just can't keep trying any more. They
are at home all day and they haven't got the natural
executive processing to get them from home to the
job centre to fill in the forms that they need to get the
interviews. It is such hard work that they just give up
and that is when they start a descent into the wacky
baccy and the rest of it. That is why we keep trying on
the job front even though it is hard.* 🔊
Billy's mum

Alcohol

All parents of teenagers are aware of the potential problems that alcohol can cause, but, of course, when your teenager has ADHD, these problems are compounded by the other behavioural issues. A bit too much to drink and your teenager can have increased levels of aggression and become attracted to risky behaviour. There is only so much you can do unless you want to operate a permanent curfew, but you may well need to be more vigilant than other parents. If you can, enlist the support of their friends to help them to drink responsibly and continue with the framework of offering lifts home from nights out and other subtle supervision for as long as your child seems to need it.

Relationships

As teenagers with ADHD often tend to be immature compared with their peers, relationships with the opposite sex may not be a factor until their late teens. The good news is that many parents report that when a steady relationship does happen, it really is a steadying influence, even on young lives that have been quite chaotic up to that point.

The future

In the area of research into ADHD these are exciting times. Understanding of causes, prevention and treatment is expanding as we find out more about genetics, behavioural science and the workings of the brain. Worldwide research is producing many promising new strands. Research in the US may help scientists to link variations in genes to differences in how people respond to ADHD medication, and research continues to look for the biological basis of ADHD and how differences in genes and brain structure and function may combine with life experiences to produce the disorder.

Let's end on an optimistic note, with a word from Hugh, a boy with a zest for life that exemplifies the best things about ADHD and a very positive attitude.

66 When the last day of school came and I thought of everything that had happened in the last year and a half, and the fact that I actually wanted to go to university and go on learning, I realised that I have a lot to thank the diagnosis and the medication for. 99

Hugh

Where to get help

Adders
www.adders.org – a website with a range of information on ADHD and the aim of promoting awareness of ADHD; provides help and information for those with the condition and their families.

ADDISS (The National Attention Deficit Disorder Information and Support Service)
Premier House, 112 Station Road, Edgware, Middlesex HA8 7BJ; 020 8952 2800; www.addiss.co.uk – a charity offering information and support for parents and professionals; provides inset training for schools and local education authorities.

Auditory integration Training Services
www.auditoryintegration.net

Barnardo's
www.barnardos.org.uk/adhdservices

British Association for Behavioural and Cognitive Psychotherapies
www.babcp.com

British Association for Counselling and Psychotherapy (BACP)
www.bacp.co.uk

British Association for Music Therapy
020 7837 6100; www.bamt.org

British Association of Nutritional Therapists
0870 606 1284; www.bant.org.uk – this organisation can help you find a qualified nutritionist in your area.

Contact a family
Helpline 0808 808 3555; www.cafamily.org.uk – a national charity supporting families who have children with different special needs and disabilities. Links with over 500 support and self-

help groups. Parents can be put in touch with a support group or another family whose child has similar problems.

DfES (Department for Education and Skills)
www.dfes.gov.uk – provides the Special Educational Needs Code of Practice.

DirectGov
www.directgov.uk – will direct you towards your local services and your nearest local authority children's centres, where a lot of courses are based. It is also the place to find details on SEN provision and statementing – National Parent Partnership Network.

Familylives.org.uk
A national charity providing help and support in all aspects of family life. It has a 24-hour parent helpline (0808 800 2222), which also gives information on Parentline plus courses.

IPSEA (Independent Parental Special Education Advice)
0800 0184016; www.ipsea.org.uk – an organisation defending children's right to special educational provision.

Learning Assessment and Neurocare Centre
www.lanc.uk.com; 01403 240002 – provides assessment and ongoing management for ADHD and similar problems either through the NHS or privately.

Listening Centre
01273 474877; www.listeningcentre.co.uk – offers assessment and 'listening therapy' to people with auditory processing problems.

Mind
15–19 Broadway, Stratford, London E15 4BQ; 0845 766 0163; www. mind.org.uk.

National Parent Partnership Network
A network supporting parents and carers of children with SEN. Contact through your local authority. The network can put you

in touch with an independent parental supporter, a trained volunteer who can help you through the statementing maze.

NICE (National Institute for Health and Clinical Excellence)

www.nice.org.uk – an independent organisation responsible for providing national guidance on promoting good health and preventing and treating ill health. The guideline on ADHD can be consulted online and covers recommendations for diagnosis and treatment options:

Attention deficit hyperactivity disorder: Diagnosis and management of ADHD in children, young people and adults. Clinical Guideline 72. London: British Psychological Society and Royal College of Psychiatrists, 2009, www.nice.org.uk/CG72.

The following NICE study is also worth a read:
Focus Group Study of Children and Young People's Experience of Psychostimulant Medication. Perceptions, knowledge and attitudes towards psychostimulant stimulant medication for ADHD: a focus group study of children and young people diagnosed with ADHD. Dr Ilina Singh, London School of Economics and Political Science; Sinead Keenan, London School of Economics and Political Science; Dr Alex Mears Healthcare Commission 2007. Available at www. nice.org.uk/nicemedia/live/12061/42064/42064.pdf.

Osteopathic Centre for Children

020 8875 5290; www.occ.uk.com

PALS (Patients Advice and Liaison Service)

www.pals.nhs.uk

Parent Partnership Services (PPS)

Statutory services offering information advice and support to parents and carers of children and young people with SEN. PPS can put parents in touch with other local and national organisations.

Sibs

Meadowfield, Oxenhope, West Yorkshire, BD22 9JD; 01535 645 453; www.sibs.org.uk – the only UK charity representing the needs of siblings of disabled people.

Special Educational Needs and Disability Tribunal

www.sendist.gov.uk

United Kingdom Council for Psychotherapy (UKCP)

www.psychotherapy.co.uk

Volunteer Reading Help

www.vrh.org.uk – an organisation that sends volunteer tutors into primary and junior schools in some areas to help with reading.

www.netmums.com

An online parenting organisation – a family of local sites that cover the UK.

www.nordoff-robbins.org.uk

020 7267 4496; a music charity dedicated to transforming the lines of vulnerable children and adults.

www.parentchannel.tv

A website supporting parents' day-to-day concerns through a collection of short videos.

www.parentinguk.org

A website directing to other sources of help; gives details of parenting classes nationwide.

YoungMinds

PO Box 52735, London EC1P 1YY, 0800 018 2138; www.youngminds.org.uk – a free, confidential telephone service providing information and advice to any adult with concerns about the mental health of a child or young person.

Index

18091958R00093

Made in the USA
Middletown, DE
26 February 2015